EDITION **6**

HESI

ADMISSION ASSESSMENT
Exam Review

EDITOR
John Lane, RT(R)(CT), BS, DC
Technologist
Radiography, Computed Tomography
The American Registry of Radiologic Technologists (ARRT)
St. Louis, Missouri

ELSEVIER

Elsevier
3251 Riverport Lane
St. Louis, Missouri 63043

Notice

Practitioners and researchers must always rely on their own experience and knowledge in evaluating and using any information, methods, compounds or experiments described herein. Because of rapid advances in the medical sciences, in particular, independent verification of diagnoses and drug dosages should be made. To the fullest extent of the law, no responsibility is assumed by Elsevier, authors, editors or contributors for any injury and/or damage to persons or property as a matter of products liability, negligence or otherwise, or from any use or operation of any methods, products, instructions, or ideas contained in the material herein.

Previous editions copyrighted 2021, 2017, 2013, 2009, and 2004.

Content Strategist: Heather D. Bays-Petrovic
Senior Content Development Specialist: Elizabeth McCormac
Publishing Services Manager: Deepthi Unni
Project Manager: Sheik Mohideen K
Book Designer: Ryan Cook

Printed in India

Last digit is the print number: 9 8 7 6 5 4 3 2 1

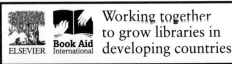

CONTRIBUTING AUTHORS

Lisa Aberle, MSRS, RT(R)(CV)
Radiography Educator
Continuing Education
Achieve RT Media
Chatsworth, Illinois

Peter J. Carpico, Med, BS
Professor of Chemistry
Stark State College
North Canton, Ohio

PREFACE

Congratulations on purchasing the *HESI Admission Assessment Exam Review*! This study guide was developed based on the HESI Admission Assessment Exam; however, test items on the HESI Admission Assessment Exam are not specifically derived from this study guide. The content in this study guide provides an overview of the subjects tested on the Admission Assessment Exam and is designed to assist students in preparation for entrance into higher education in a variety of health-related professions. The *HESI Admission Assessment Exam Review* is written at the high school and beginning college levels and offers the basic knowledge that is necessary to be successful on the Admission Assessment Exam.

The HESI Admission Assessment Exam consists of 10 different exams—eight academically oriented exams and two personally oriented exams. The academically oriented subjects consist of:

- Mathematics
- Reading Comprehension
- Vocabulary
- Grammar
- Biology
- Chemistry
- Anatomy and Physiology

Chapter content in the *HESI Admission Assessment Exam Review* includes conversion tables and practice problems in the Mathematics chapter; step-by-step explanations in the Reading Comprehension and Grammar chapters; a substantial list of words used in health professions in the Vocabulary chapter; rationales and sample questions in the Biology and Chemistry chapters; and helpful terminology in the Anatomy and Physiology chapter. Also included throughout the exam review are "HESI Hint" boxes, which are designed to offer students a suggestion, an example, or a reminder pertaining to a specific topic.

The personally oriented exams consist of a Learning Style assessment and a Personality Profile. These exams are intended to offer students insights into their study habits, learning preferences, and dispositions relating to academic achievement. Students generally like to take these personally oriented exams for the purpose of personal insight and discussion. Because each of these exams takes only approximately 15 minutes to complete, the school may include them in their administration of the Admission Assessment Exam.

Schools can choose to administer any one, or all, of these exams provided by the Admission Assessment. For example, programs that do not require biology, chemistry, or anatomy and physiology for entry would not administer those specific Admission Assessment science-oriented exams.

The HESI Admission Assessment Exam has been used by colleges, universities, and health-related institutions as part of the selection and placement process for applicants and newly admitted students for approximately 10 years.

Study Hints

It is always a good idea to prepare for any exam. When you begin to study for the Admission Assessment Exam, make sure you allocate adequate time and do not feel rushed. Set up a schedule that provides an hour or two each day to review material in the *HESI Admission Assessment Exam Review*. Mark the time you set aside on a calendar to remind yourself when to study each day. Before you begin, take the 25-question Pretest at the beginning of the text to help you initially assess your strengths and weaknesses of the content. For each section in the *HESI Admission Assessment Exam Review*, review the material that is relevant to your particular field of the health-care professions. Complete the review questions at the end of each chapter, then complete the 50-question Posttest at the end of the text. This Posttest gives you additional practice in the text's subject areas using a more comprehensive approach. The Posttest will help you to assess your readiness for the exam. Once you have completed your review and self-assessment of topics in the study guide, more test-taking practice is available on the text's corresponding Evolve site (http://www.elsevier.com/HESI/A2Review) with two comprehensive 82-question Practice Exams on the various subject areas that will help you prepare for the Admissions Assessment Exam. If you are having trouble with the review questions or the Practice Exams for a particular section, review that content in the *HESI Admission Assessment Exam Review* study guide again. It may also be helpful to go back to your textbook and class notes for additional review.

Test-Taking Hints

1. Read each question carefully and completely. Make sure you understand what the question is asking.
2. Identify the key words or phrases in the question. These words or phrases will provide critical information about how to answer the question.
3. Rephrase the question in your words.
   A. Ask yourself, "What is the question really asking?"
   B. Eliminate nonessential information from the question.
   C. Sometimes writers use terminology that may be unfamiliar to you. Do not be confused by a new writing style.
4. Rule out options (if they are presented).
   A. Read all of the responses completely.
   B. Rule out any options that are clearly incorrect.
   C. Mentally mark through incorrect options in your head.
   D. Differentiate between the remaining options, considering your knowledge of the subject.
5. Computer tests do not allow an option for skipping questions and returning to them later. Practice answering every question as it appears.

Do not second-guess yourself. TRUST YOUR ANSWERS.

TABLE OF CONTENTS

1. Change $6\frac{1}{3}$ to an improper fraction.
  A. $\frac{6}{3}$
  B. $\frac{10}{3}$
  C. $\frac{19}{3}$
  D. $\frac{24}{3}$

2. Which word means the same as the underlined word in the sentence?
Many stores in town have closed due to the <u>long-lasting</u> shortage of workers.
  A. Gratuitous
  B. Impending
  C. Precipitous
  D. Chronic

3. In the hierarchical system for naming organisms, which category is the largest?
  A. Kingdom
  B. Class
  C. Genus
  D. Species

4. Through which structure does urine leave the body?
  A. Ureter
  B. Urethra
  C. Bladder
  D. Renal tubule

5. The mass of a golf ball is 0.045 kg. What is this number in scientific notation?
  A. 4.5×10^{-2} kg
  B. 4.5×10^{-3} kg
  C. 45×10^{-3} kg
  D. 45×10^{-2} kg

6. Find the value of y:
  $$-25 \times y = -100$$
  A. 4
  B. -75

C. -4
D. 75

Use the passage below to answer questions 7–9.

Penicillin

Antibiotics are among the most commonly prescribed drugs today. Before the discovery of the first antibiotic, there was no effective treatment for pneumonia or other bacterial infections. Until antibiotics were available, even a small cut on the surface of the skin could result in a potentially grave infection.

The world's first true antibiotic was discovered by a professor of bacteriology named Alexander Fleming. In 1928, Fleming was performing experiments with staphylococcal bacteria. Fleming noticed that the bacteria in one of his Petri dishes was dying. Unlike the other samples, this dish had become contaminated by mold spores. Fleming was able to identify the mold as a member of the *Penicillium* genus.

When Fleming grew this mold in a pure culture, he found that it produced a substance that was effective against all gram-positive pathogens. He would eventually refer to this "mold juice" as penicillin. Fleming admitted that his discovery was purely accidental, but his groundbreaking work in developing the first antibiotic revolutionized medicine and saved millions of lives.

7. What is the author's primary purpose in writing this essay?
  A. To explain how penicillin was discovered.
  B. To warn about the dangers of bacterial infections.
  C. To inform readers about the life of a famous inventor.
  D. To promote the use of antibiotics to treat bacterial infections.

8. According to the passage, which statement is false?
   A. Fleming discovered penicillin by accident.
   B. Fleming discovered the first true antibiotic.
   C. Penicillin is effective against gram-positive pathogens.
   D. One of Fleming's Petri dishes became contaminated with bacteria.

9. What is the meaning of the word *grave* in the first paragraph?
   A. Severe
   B. Mild
   C. Hidden
   D. Obvious

10. Which word means the same as the underlined word in the sentence?
    Rubbing your eyes too much might <u>harm</u> your vison.
    A. Impede
    B. Impair
    C. Impinge
    D. Impact

11. Which word in the following sentence is a preposition?
    Mom and dad always remind us to be home before dark.
    A. Always
    B. Us
    C. To
    D. Before

12. Twelve (12) more than a number is five (5). What is the number?
    A. −7
    B. 7
    C. −17
    D. 17

13. Select the best word for the blank in the following sentence.
    I must remember to _____ my book to class today.
    A. Bring
    B. Take
    C. Brought
    D. Took

14. Which subatomic particles carry a positive charge?
    A. Protons and electrons
    B. Protons only
    C. Neutrons and electrons
    D. Neutrons only

15. If a DNA strand has a base sequence GTACGT, what is the sequence of the complementary segment of DNA?
    A. GTACGT
    B. CATGCA
    C. TGCATG
    D. ACGTAC

16. Which word in the following sentence is the direct object?
    Tom's dad gave him a bicycle for his birthday.
    A. Dad
    B. Him
    C. Bicycle
    D. Birthday

17. Which property of water explains why the oceans are helpful in stabilizing the climate?
    A. Water molecules spread apart in freezing temperatures.
    B. Water has strong cohesive and adhesive properties.
    C. Water can act as both an acid and a base.
    D. Water has a relatively high specific heat value.

18. Select the meaning of the underlined word in the sentence.
    The negotiator offered a peaceful solution to the <u>perpetual</u> conflict between the two nations.
    A. Constant
    B. Serious
    C. Recent
    D. Minor

19. Multiply: 128×313
    A. 37,944
    B. 38,044
    C. 40,164
    D. 40,064

20. Which of the following sentences is grammatically correct?
    A. It's raining outside, and I can't find my umbrella.
    B. It's raining outside and I can't find my umbrella.
    C. It's raining outside, I can't find my umbrella.
    D. It's raining outside I can't find my umbrella.

21. Which function is performed by the gallbladder?
    A. Protein digestion
    B. Blood filtration
    C. Bile storage
    D. Insulin secretion

22. Which biomolecules are composed of amino acids?
    A. Carbohydrates
    B. Lipids
    C. Proteins
    D. Nucleic acids

23. Find the mean for the following set of numbers:
    {6, 6, 17, 53, 63}
    A. 5
    B. 6
    C. 17
    D. 29

24. Which is a function of smooth muscle tissue?
    A. Produces involuntary movements of the organs.
    B. Regulates the pumping action of the heart.
    C. Initiates and conducts nerve impulses.
    D. Secretes enzymes and hormones.

25. Which word means the same as the underlined word in the sentence?
    The judge would not allow the witness to testify despite <u>myriad</u> objections from the defense team.
    A. False
    B. Numerous
    C. Angry
    D. Loud

ANSWERS TO PRETEST

1. C—To change $6\frac{1}{3}$ into an improper fraction, multiply the denominator (3) by 6 and add 1, then place this value (19) over the denominator:
   $3 \times 6 + 1 = 19$
   Answer: $^{19}/_3$

2. D—*Chronic* means "long-lasting."

3. A—In the hierarchic organizational system for nomenclature, kingdom is the largest and most inclusive category.

4. B—Urine is transported from the bladder to outside the body through the urethra.

5. A—To convert from standard notation to scientific notation ($N \times 10^{power}$), rewrite the significant figures with one digit in front of the decimal point and the rest of the digits after the decimal point (N must be at least 1 and less than 10):
   0.045 kg → 4.5
   Count the number of places you moved the decimal point to convert the original number to the new number. This number (2) becomes the exponent. If you moved the decimal point to the right to get the new number, the exponent is negative:

   $0.045 \text{ kg} = 4.5 \times 10^{-2} \text{ kg}$

6. A—Solve: $-25 \times y = -100$
   Isolate the variable (divide both sides by −25):
   $$\frac{-25 \times y}{-25} = \frac{-100}{-25}$$
   $y = 4$

7. A—Most of the information in the passage describes Alexander Fleming's accidental discovery of penicillin. The author's primary purpose is to explain how penicillin was discovered.

8. D—The passage states that Fleming's Petri dish became contaminated with mold spores, not bacteria.

9. A—The passage states that "even a small cut…could result in a potentially *grave* infection." In this context, the word *small* can be taken to mean "harmless," which is an antonym of the word in question. This clue should help the reader understand that *grave* means "severe."

10. B—*Impair* means "to harm or damage."

11. D—Prepositions can be used to express relations in time. In the sentence *Mom and dad always remind us to be home before dark*, the preposition *before* indicates that one thing (being home) must occur before something else (dark).

12. A—Rewrite the word problem as an equation ($n + 12 = 5$), then isolate the variable (subtract 12 from both sides):
$n + 12 - 12 = 5 - 12$
$n = -7$

13. B—In this sentence, the action is away from the speaker, who will carry the book from a near place (where the speaker is) to a far place (the classroom). Therefore, the correct word is "take."

14. B—Two types of subatomic particles carry a charge, but only protons carry a positive electrical charge.

15. B—Base pairing rules for writing complimentary DNA strands are as follows: guanine (G) ↔ cytosine (C), adenine (A) ↔ thymine (T). The complementary DNA sequence for GTACGT is CATGCA.

16. C—The direct object is the word that is directly affected by the action of the verb. In this sentence, the noun "bicycle" receives the action of the verb "gave."

17. D—Water has a relatively high specific heat due to the hydrogen bonds between water molecules; this property allows water to resist shifts in temperature. One benefit of high specific heat is the ability of oceans or large bodies of water to stabilize climates.

18. A—*Perpetual* means "constant" or "nonstop."

19. D—Multiply: $128 \times 313 =$
```
    128
×   313
    384 (128 × 3)
   1280 (128 × 10)
 38,400 (128 × 300)
 40,064
```

20. A—When two or more independent clauses are separated by a coordinating conjunction, a comma is needed before the conjunction. In this sentence, a comma is needed before the coordinating conjunction "and."

21. C—The gall bladder is a digestive organ located under the liver that stores bile before releasing it into the small intestine.

22. C—Amino acids are joined together to make proteins.

23. D—The mean, or average, is equal to the sum of all the values of a data set divided by the total number of values. The mean of the following data set is 29:
{6, 6, 17, 53, 63}
$6 + 6 + 17 + 53 + 63 = 145$
$145 \div 5 = 29$

24. A—Smooth muscles line the walls of blood vessels and hollow organs and produce involuntary movements of the organs.

25. B—*Myriad* means "numerous" or "great in number."

MATHEMATICS

1

Members of the health professions use math every day to calculate medication dosage, nutritional needs, intravenous drip rates, fluid intake and output, and a host of other measures related to patient care. Safe and effective care is the goal of all who work in health professions. Therefore, it is essential that students entering the health professions understand and make calculations using whole numbers, fractions, decimals, and percentages.

The purpose of this chapter is to review the addition, subtraction, multiplication, and division of whole numbers, fractions, decimals, and percentages. Measures of central tendency and basic algebra will also be reviewed. Mastery of these basic mathematic functions is an integral step toward a career in the health professions.

CHAPTER OUTLINE

Basic Addition and Subtraction
Basic Multiplication (Whole Numbers)
Basic Division (Whole Numbers)
Decimals
Fractions

Addition of Fractions
Subtraction of Fractions
Multiplication of Fractions
Division of Fractions
Changing Fractions to Decimals
Changing Decimals to Fractions

Ratios and Proportions
Percentages
Mean, Median, and Mode
Algebra
Other Helpful Information
Answers to Sample Problems

KEY TERMS

Common Denominator
Constant
Denominator
Digit
Dividend
Divisor
Exponent
Expression
Factor

Fraction Bar
Improper Fraction
Least Common Denominator
Mean, Median, and Mode
Mixed Number
Numerator
Percent
Place Value
Product

Proper Fraction
Proportion
Quotient
Ratio
Reciprocals
Remainder
Terminating Decimal
Variable

Basic Addition and Subtraction

Digit: Any number 1 through 9 and 0 (e.g., the number 7 is a digit)
Place Value: The value of the position of a digit in a number (e.g., in the number 321, the number 2 is in the "tens" position)

$$
\begin{array}{ccc}
\text{Hundreds} & \text{Tens} & \text{Units (ones)} \\
| & | & | \\
\hline
3 & 2 & 1
\end{array}
$$

HESI Hint

1 ten = 10 ones
1 hundred = 100 ones
1 thousand = 1000 ones

Basic Addition

Example 1

382 + 212

$$
\begin{array}{r}
382 \\
+\ 212 \\
\hline
594
\end{array}
$$

Steps

1. Line up the **digits** according to **place value.**
2. Add the digits starting from right to left.
   - Ones: $2 + 2 = 4$
   - Tens: $8 + 1 = 9$
   - Hundreds: $3 + 2 = 5$

Addition with Regrouping

HESI Hint

To solve an addition problem, it may be necessary to regroup by moving, or carrying over, an extra digit from one place value column to the next.

Example 2

748 + 523

$$
\begin{array}{r}
\overset{1}{7}48 \\
+\ 523 \\
\hline
1{,}271
\end{array}
$$

Steps

1. Line up the digits according to place value.
2. Add:
   - Ones: $8 + 3 = 11$
   - Carry the 1 to the tens place, which is one place to the left.
   - Tens: $1 + 4 + 2 = 7$
   - Hundreds: $7 + 5 = 12$

Basic Subtraction

Subtraction provides the difference between two numbers.

HESI Hint

It may be easier to solve a subtraction problem by first rewriting it vertically.

Example 1

$3,884 - 1,671$

$$
\begin{array}{r}
3,884 \\
- 1,671 \\
\hline
2,213
\end{array}
$$

Steps

1. Line up the digits according to place value.
2. Subtract:
   - Ones: $4 - 1 = 3$
   - Tens: $8 - 7 = 1$
   - Hundreds: $8 - 6 = 2$
   - Thousands: $3 - 1 = 2$

Subtraction with Regrouping

HESI Hint

Remember, if the number to subtract is not a positive number, you must borrow or regroup from one place value to a lower place value.

Example 1

$862 - 57$

$$
\begin{array}{r}
\overset{5\ \ 12}{8\,\cancel{6}\,\cancel{2}} \\
- 5\,7 \\
\hline
8\,0\,5
\end{array}
$$

Steps

1. Align the digits according to place value.

2. Subtract:
   - Ones: $12 - 7 = 5$
   - Tens: $5 - 5 = 0$
   - Hundreds: $8 - 0 = 8$

SAMPLE PROBLEMS

Add or subtract each of the following problems as indicated.
1. $1{,}786 + 257 =$
2. $273 + 47 =$
3. $1{,}644 + 357 =$
4. $73 + 211 + 22 =$
5. $382 - 150 =$
6. $246 - 47 =$
7. $6{,}640 - 518 =$
8. $17{,}444 - 923 =$
9. Sam walks 2 blocks to Stacey's house. They both walk 5 blocks to the park. How many blocks has Sam walked?
10. Lisa buys 12 eggs from the store so she can make pancakes. The pancake recipe calls for 3 eggs. How many eggs will Lisa have left after making the pancakes?

Basic Multiplication (Whole Numbers)

The process of multiplication is essentially repeated addition.
Product: The answer to a multiplication problem.

HESI Hint

Remember, the zero is used as a placeholder to keep the problem aligned. If you do not skip a space, the answer will be incorrect. Below is an example of a well-aligned problem.

$$
\begin{array}{r}
24571 \\
\times\ 1233 \\
\hline
73{,}713 \\
737{,}130 \\
4{,}914{,}200 \\
+\ 24{,}571{,}000 \\
\hline
30{,}296{,}043
\end{array}
\begin{array}{l}
\\
\\
\rightarrow \text{Ones} \\
\rightarrow \text{Tens} \\
\rightarrow \text{Hundreds} \\
\rightarrow \text{Thousands} \\
\end{array}
$$

Example 1

18×4

$$
\begin{array}{r}
\overset{3}{1}8 \\
\times\ 4 \\
\hline
72
\end{array}
$$

Steps

1. Multiply one digit at a time.
   - Ones: $4 \times 8 = 32$

   Carry the 3 to the tens place, and write the 2 in the ones place.
   - Tens: $4 \times 1 = 4$
2. Remember that 3 was carried over from 32. Add 3 and 4, then write 7 in the tens place.

Example 2

713×24

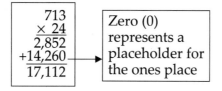

$$\begin{array}{r} 713 \\ \times\ 24 \\ \hline 2,852 \\ +14,260 \\ \hline 17,112 \end{array}$$

Zero (0) represents a placeholder for the ones place

Steps

1. Multiply 713×24.
   - $4 \times 3 = 12$
   - $4 \times 1 = 4 + 1 = 5$
   - $4 \times 7 = 28$
2. Multiply 713×2 (remember to line up the ones digit with the 4 by using zero as a placeholder).
   - $2 \times 3 = 6$
   - $2 \times 1 = 2$
   - $2 \times 7 = 14$
3. Add the two products together.
   - $2,852 + 14,260 = 17,112$ (the final product)

Example 3

411×242

$$\begin{array}{r} 411 \\ \times\ 242 \\ \hline 822 \\ 16,440 \\ +\ 82,200 \\ \hline 99,462 \end{array}$$

Steps

1. Multiply 411×2.
   - $2 \times 1 = 2$
   - $2 \times 1 = 2$
   - $2 \times 4 = 8$
2. Multiply 411×4.
   - $4 \times 1 = 4$ (remember to use a zero for a placeholder)
   - $4 \times 1 = 4$
   - $4 \times 4 = 16$

3. Multiply 411×2.
   - $2 \times 1 = 2$
   - $2 \times 1 = 2$
   - $2 \times 4 = 8$
4. Add the three products together.
   - $822 + 16,440 + 82,200 = 99,462$ (the final product)

SAMPLE PROBLEMS

Multiply.

1. $57 \times 36 =$
2. $63 \times 73 =$
3. $821 \times 22 =$
4. $529 \times 47 =$
5. $954 \times 75 =$
6. $262 \times 94 =$
7. $123 \times 529 =$
8. $2,943 \times 293 =$
9. It takes 18 man-hours for an automobile factory to build a car. How many man-hours does it take to build 92 cars?
10. A bakery sells boxes of donuts with 13 donuts in each box. If the bakery sells 52 boxes of donuts, how many total donuts were sold?

Basic Division (Whole Numbers)

Dividend: The number being divided.
Divisor: The number by which the dividend is divided.
Quotient: The answer to a division problem.
Remainder: The portion of the dividend that is not evenly divisible by the divisor.

HESI Hint

$$5\overline{)45} = 9$$

The 45 represents the **dividend** (the number being divided), the 5 represents the **divisor** (the number by which the dividend is divided), and the 9 represents the **quotient** (the answer to the division problem). It is best not to leave a division problem with a **remainder**, but to end it as a fraction or decimal instead. To make the problem into a decimal, add a decimal point and zeros at the end of the dividend and continue. If a remainder continues to occur, round to the hundredths place.

Example
$233.547 \rightarrow 233.55$ (the 7 rounds the 4 to a 5)

Example 1
$42 \div 7$

$$7\overline{)42} = 6$$
$$-42$$
$$\overline{0}$$

Steps

1. Set up the problem.
2. Use a series of multiplication and subtraction problems to solve a division problem.
3. $7 \times ? = 42$
   - Multiply: $7 \times 6 = 42$
   - Subtract: $42 - 42 = 0$
   - The quotient (or answer) is 6.

Example 2

$464 \div 4$

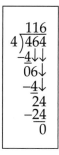

Steps

1. Set up the problem.
2. Begin with the hundreds place.
   - $4 \times ? = 4$. We know $4 \times 1 = 4$; therefore, place the 1 (quotient) above the 4 in the hundreds place (dividend). Place the other 4 under the hundreds place and subtract: $4 - 4 = 0$.
   - Bring down the next number, which is 6; $4 \times ? = 6$. There is no number that can be multiplied by 4 that will equal 6 exactly, so try to get as close as possible without going over 6. Use $4 \times 1 = 4$ and set it up just like the last subtraction problem: $6 - 4 = 2$.
   - Bring down the 4 from the dividend, which results in the number 24 (the 2 came from the remainder of $6 - 4 = 2$).
   - $4 \times ? = 24$; $? = 6$. The two becomes the next number in the quotient. $24 - 24 = 0$. There is no remainder.
   - The quotient (or answer) is 116.

Example 3

$163 \div 5$

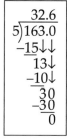

Steps

1. Set up the problem.
2. The 5 (divisor) does not divide into 1 but does divide into 16.
3. $5 \times 3 = 15$. Write the 3 in the quotient. (It is written above the 6 in 16 because that is the last digit in the number.)
   - $5 \times 3 = 15$
   - $16 - 15 = 1$
4. Bring the 3 down. Combine the 1 (remainder from $16 - 15$) and 3 to create 13.
5. The 5 does not divide evenly into 13; therefore, try to get close without going over.
   - $5 \times 2 = 10$
   - $13 - 10 = 3$
6. There is a remainder of 3, but there is no number left in the dividend. Add a decimal point and zeros and continue to divide.
7. The quotient (or answer) is 32.6 (thirty-two and six tenths).

SAMPLE PROBLEMS

Divide.

1. $51 \div 4 =$
2. $6,400 \div 8 =$
3. $3,732 \div 2 =$
4. $357 \div 17 =$
5. $4,725 \div 9 =$
6. $2,925 \div 3 =$
7. $787 \div 8 =$
8. $6,281 \div 5 =$
9. There are 72 bottles of water for a soccer team with 16 players. If each player receives the same amount of water, how many bottles of water can each player have?
10. Tim is driving 270 miles to visit his parents. Tim's car can travel 18 miles on 1 gallon of gas. How many gallons of gas does Tim need to make it to his parents' house?

Decimals

A decimal pertains to tenths or to the number 10.

Place value: Regarding decimals, numbers to the right of the decimal point have different terms from the whole numbers to the left of the decimal point. Each digit in a number occupies a position called a **place value.**

Addition and Subtraction of Decimals

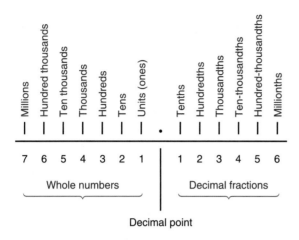

HESI Hint

Remember, whole numbers are written to the left of the decimal point and place values are written to the right of the decimal point. Line the numbers up vertically before solving the problem.

HESI Hint

The word "and" stands for the decimal when writing a number in words.
Example: 5.7 (five *and* seven tenths)

Example 1

$1.3 + 7.2$

$$
\begin{array}{r}
1.3 \\
+\ 7.2 \\
\hline
8.5
\end{array}
$$

Steps

1. Align the decimal points.
2. Add the tenths together: $3 + 2 = 5$
3. Add the ones together: $1 + 7 = 8$
4. Final answer: 8.5 (eight and five tenths).

Example 2

$6 + 22.13$

$$
\begin{array}{r}
22.13 \\
+\ 6.00 \\
\hline
28.13
\end{array}
$$

Steps

1. Align the decimal points.

- It might be difficult to align the 6 because it does not have a decimal point.
- Remember that after the ones place, there is a decimal point. To help with organization, add zeros (placeholders). **Example:** $6 = 6.00$

2. Add the hundredths: $3 + 0 = 3$
3. Add the tenths: $1 + 0 = 1$
4. Add the ones: $2 + 6 = 8$
5. Add the tens: $2 + 0 = 2$
6. Final answer: 28.13 (twenty-eight and thirteen hundredths).

Example 3

$9.46 - 7.34$

$$\begin{array}{r} 9.46 \\ -\ 7.34 \\ \hline 2.12 \end{array}$$

Steps

1. Align the decimal points.
2. Subtract the hundredths: $6 - 4 = 2$
3. Subtract the tenths: $4 - 3 = 1$
4. Subtract the ones: $9 - 7 = 2$
5. Final answer: 2.12 (two and twelve hundredths).

Example 4

$22 - 7.99$

$$\begin{array}{r} {}^{1}\ \ {}^{9\ 10} \\ 2\,\cancel{2}\,.\cancel{0}\cancel{0} \\ -7.9\cancel{9} \\ \hline 14.01 \end{array}$$

Steps

1. Align the decimal points.
2. Because 22 is a whole number, add a decimal point and zeros.
3. $0.00 - 0.99$ cannot be subtracted; therefore, 1 must be borrowed from the 22 and regrouped.
4. The 2 in the ones place becomes 1, the 0 in the tenths place becomes 9, and the 0 in the hundredths place becomes 10.
5. Subtract the hundredths: $10 - 9 = 1$
6. Subtract the tenths: $9 - 9 = 0$
7. Subtract the ones: $21 - 7 = 14$
   - 1 was borrowed from the tens in order to subtract the 7.
8. Final answer: 14.01 (fourteen and one hundredth).

Solve each of the following decimal problems as indicated.
1. $3.12 + 6.7 =$
2. $8.725 + 41.72 =$
3. $127.2 + 83 =$
4. $43 + 9.57 =$
5. $4.6 + 3.66 + 11 =$
6. $22 - 14.18 =$
7. $67.74 - 9.83 =$
8. $17.56 - 9.88 =$
9. Robin used the company car for 3 business trips. She traveled 3.2 miles on Monday, 4.75 miles on Wednesday, and 7.3 miles on Friday. How many total miles did Robin travel for the week?
10. A dressmaker needs 4.25 yards of fabric to make a blue dress, but only 2.5 yards of blue fabric are left in stock. How many additional yards of fabric does the dressmaker need to complete the dress?

Multiplication of Decimals

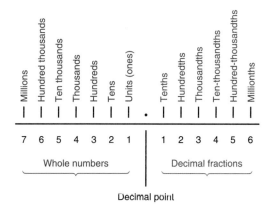

Example 1

81.2×4.2

$$
\begin{array}{r}
81.2 \\
\times\ 4.2 \\
\hline
1624 \\
+\ 32480 \\
\hline
341.04
\end{array}
$$

1 decimal place
+ 1 decimal place
2 decimal places

Move the decimal point two places to the left in the final product.

Steps

1. Multiply 812×42 (do not worry about the decimal point until the final product has been calculated).

2. Starting from the right, count the decimal places in both numbers and add together (two decimal places).
3. Move to the left two places, and then place the decimal point.

Example 2

0.002×3.4

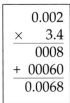

0.002	3 decimal places
$\times$ 3.4	+ 1 decimal place
0008	4 decimal places
+ 00060	Move four places to the left.
0.0068	

Steps

1. Multiply 2×34.
2. Starting from the right, count the decimal places in both numbers and add together (four decimal places).
3. Move to the left four places, and then place the decimal.

Example 3

8.23×3

8.23	2 decimal places
$\times$ 3	+ 0 decimal places
24.69	2 decimal places
	Move two places to the left.

Steps

1. Multiply 823×3.
2. Starting from the right, count the decimal places in both numbers and add together (two decimal places).
3. Move to the left two places, and then place the decimal point.

SAMPLE PROBLEMS

Multiply the decimals in the following problems as indicated.
1. $0.9 \times 4.53 =$
2. $31.22 \times 7 =$
3. $4.04 \times 6.1 =$
4. $321.1 \times 18 =$
5. $0.9112 \times 8.13 =$
6. $21.2 \times 7 =$
7. $0.009 \times 45.2 =$
8. $245.24 \times .003 =$
9. Tina's water bottle holds 24.6 ounces of liquid. If Tina drinks 2.5 bottles of water, how much water has she drunk?
10. Dennis walks 1.2 miles to the store to buy groceries. He walks another 1.2 miles to bring the groceries home. How many miles does Dennis have to walk to complete 2 grocery trips?

Division of Decimals

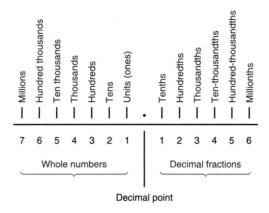

Example 1

$48 \div 2.5$

$$
\begin{array}{r}
19.2 \\
2.\underline{5} \overline{)\, 48.\underline{0}.0} \\
-25 \downarrow\downarrow \\
\overline{230\downarrow} \\
-225\downarrow \\
\overline{50} \\
-50 \\
\overline{0}
\end{array}
$$

Steps

1. Set up the division problem.
2. Move the decimal point in 2.5 one place to the right, making it a whole number.
3. What is done to one side must be done to the other side. Move the decimal point one place to the right in 48, making it 480, and then bring the decimal point up into the quotient.
4. Divide normally.
   - $25 \times 1 = 25$
   - Subtract: $48 - 25 = 23$
   - Bring down the zero to make 230.
   - $25 \times 9 = 225$. This is as close to 230 as possible without going over.
   - Subtract: $230 - 225 = 5$
   - Add a zero to the dividend and bring it down to the 5, making it 50.
   - $25 \times 2 = 50$
   - $50 - 50 = 0$
5. The quotient is 19.2.

Example 2

2.468 ÷ 0.2

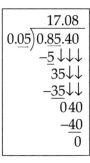

```
        12.34
0.2)2.4.68
    −2
     04
    −4
     06
     −6
      08
     −8
      0
```

Steps

1. Set up the division problem.
2. Move the decimal point in the divisor one place to the right, making it a whole number (2).
3. Move the decimal point one place to the right in the dividend, changing 2.468 to 24.68. Bring the decimal point up into the quotient.
4. Divide normally.

Example 3

0.854 ÷ 0.05

```
          17.08
0.05)0.85.40
     −5↓↓↓
      35↓↓
     −35↓↓
       040
       −40
         0
```

Steps

1. Set up the division problem.
2. Move the decimal point in the divisor two places to the right, making it a whole number.
3. Move the decimal point two places to the right in the dividend, changing 0.854 into 85.4. Bring the decimal point up into the quotient.
4. Divide normally.

SAMPLE PROBLEMS

Divide the decimals in the following problems as indicated.

1. 28.2 ÷ 0.6 =
2. 73.25 ÷ 0.25 =
3. 65.6 ÷ 0.8 =
4. 43.54 ÷ 0.7 =

5. $5.202 \div 0.45 =$

6. $912 \div 0.2 =$

7. $0.052 \div 0.8 =$

8. $0.624 \div 0.26 =$

9. Dan's pie crust recipe calls for 1.25 ounces of canola oil per crust. How many pie crusts can Dan make if he has 10 ounces of canola oil?

10. A carpenter is cutting a board to make shelves for a bookcase. The board is 2.44 meters long, and each shelf will be 0.61 meters long. How many shelves will the bookcase have?

Fractions

In mathematics, a fraction is a way to express a part in relation to the total.

Numerator: The top number in a fraction.

Denominator: The bottom number in a fraction.

Fraction Bar: The line between the numerator and denominator. The bar is another symbol for division.

Factor: A number that divides evenly into another number.

Least Common Denominator (LCD): The smallest multiple that two numbers share.

Improper Fraction: A fraction where the numerator is larger than the denominator.

Proper Fraction: A fraction where the denominator is larger than the numerator.

Mixed Number: A whole number combined with a proper fraction.

Common Denominator: Two or more fractions having the same denominator.

Reciprocals: Pairs of numbers that equal 1 when multiplied together.

Terminating Decimal: A decimal that is not continuous.

HESI Hint

- The **numerator** is the top number of the fraction. It represents the part or pieces.
- The **denominator** is the bottom number of the fraction. It represents the total or whole amount.
- The fraction bar is the line that separates the numerator and the denominator.

$$\frac{\text{Numerator (part)}}{\text{Denominator (whole)}} \text{ Fraction bar}$$

Reducing Fractions Using the Greatest Common Factor

A **factor** is a number that divides evenly into another number.

Factors of 12:

- $1 \times 12 = 12$
- $2 \times 6 = 12$
- $3 \times 4 = 12$

12 {1, 2, 3, 4, 6, 12}: Listing the factors helps determine the greatest common factor between two or more numbers.

$$\frac{1}{2} = \frac{2}{4}, \frac{3}{6}, \frac{4}{8}, \frac{5}{10}, \frac{6}{12}, \frac{7}{14}, \frac{8}{16}, \frac{9}{18}, \frac{10}{20}$$

All represent one-half.

Reducing fractions can also be called reducing a fraction to its lowest terms or simplest form. A fraction is reduced to the lowest terms by finding an equivalent fraction in which the numerator and denominator are as small as possible. You may need to reduce fractions to work with them in an equation or for solving a problem. When a fraction is reduced to lowest terms, there is no number (other than 1) that can be evenly divided into both the numerator and the denominator.

$$1 = \frac{1}{1}, \frac{2}{2}, \frac{3}{3}, \frac{4}{4}, \frac{5}{5}, \frac{6}{6}, \frac{7}{7}, \frac{8}{8}, \frac{9}{9}, \frac{10}{10}$$

Example 1

Reduce $\dfrac{4}{24}$

Factors of 4 and 24:

4 {1, 2, **4**}

24 {1, 2, 3, **4**, 6, 8, 12, 24}

The greatest common factor is 4; therefore, divide the numerator and denominator by 4.

$$\frac{4}{24} \div \frac{4}{4} = \frac{1}{6}$$

Example 2

Reduce $\dfrac{12}{20}$

Factors of 12 and 20:

12 {1, 2, 3, **4**, 6, 12}

20 {1, 2, **4**, 5, 10, 20}

The greatest common factor is 4 (they do have 1 and 2 in common, but the greatest factor is used to reduce to lowest terms).

$$\frac{12}{20} \div \frac{4}{4} = \frac{3}{5}$$

Least Common Denominator

The LCD is the smallest multiple that two numbers share. Determining the LCD is an essential step in the addition, subtraction, and ordering of fractions.

Example 1

Find the LCD for $\dfrac{3}{4}$ and $\dfrac{7}{9}$

Steps

1. List the multiples (multiplication tables) of each denominator.
   - 4: $4 \times 1 = 4$, $4 \times 2 = 8$, $4 \times 3 = 12$, $4 \times 4 = 16$, $4 \times 5 = 20$, $4 \times 6 = 24$, $4 \times 7 = 28$, $4 \times 8 = 32$, $4 \times 9 = 36$, $4 \times 10 = 40$
   - 4 {4, 8, 12, 16, 20, 24, 28, 32, 36, 40}—this will be the standard form throughout for listing multiples.
   - 9 {9, 18, 27, 36, 45, 54, 63, 72, 81, 90}
2. Compare each for the least common multiple.
   - 4 {4, 8, 12, 16, 20, 24, 28, 32, **36**, 40}
   - 9 {9, 18, 27, **36**, 45, 54, 63, 72, 81, 90}
3. The LCD of 4 and 9 is 36 ($4 \times 9 = 36$ and $9 \times 4 = 36$).

Example 2

Find the LCD for $\frac{1}{15}$ and $\frac{2}{3}$

Steps

1. List the multiples of each denominator, and find the common multiples.
   - 15 {**15**, 30, 45, 60, 75, 90, 105, 120, 135, 150}
   - 3 {3, 6, 9, 12, **15**, 18, 21, 24, 27, 30}
2. The LCD of 15 and 3 is 15 ($15 \times 1 = 15$ and 3×5 is 15).

Changing Improper Fractions into Mixed Numbers

An **improper fraction** occurs when the numerator is larger than the denominator. An improper fraction can be reduced and made into a mixed number.

Example

$$\frac{17}{5} \rightarrow 5\overline{)17} \begin{array}{c} 3 \\ \underline{15} \\ 2 \end{array} \rightarrow 3\frac{2}{5}$$

Steps

1. Turn an improper fraction into a mixed number by dividing. The top number (17) is the numerator; the bottom number (5) is the denominator.
2. The 3 becomes the whole number.
3. The remainder (2) becomes the numerator.
4. The denominator stays the same.

Changing Mixed Numbers into Improper Fractions

A **mixed number** is a whole number combined with a proper fraction.

Example

$$5\frac{2}{3} \rightarrow 5\frac{+2}{3} = (5 \times 3) + 2 = 17 \rightarrow \frac{17}{3}$$

Steps

1. To make a mixed number into an improper fraction, multiply the denominator (3) and whole number (5) together, then add the numerator (2).
2. Place this new numerator (17) over the denominator (3), which stays the same in the mixed number.

Addition of Fractions

Addition with Common Denominators

Example

$$\frac{1}{9} + \frac{7}{9} = \frac{8}{9}$$

Steps

1. Add the numerators together: $1 + 7 = 8$.
2. The denominator (9) stays the same. This it is called a **common denominator.**
3. Answer: $\dfrac{8}{9}$ (eight ninths).

Addition with Unlike Denominators

Example

$$\frac{1}{3} + \frac{4}{9}$$

$$\frac{1 \times 3}{3 \times 3} = \frac{3}{9}$$

$$\frac{4 \times 1}{9 \times 1} = \frac{4}{9}$$

$$\frac{3}{9} + \frac{4}{9} = \frac{7}{9}$$

Steps

1. Find the LCD by listing the multiples of each denominator.
   - 3 {3, 6, **9**, 12, 15}
   - 9 {**9**, 27, 36, 45}
   - The LCD is 9.
2. Rename the fraction(s) with the new (common) denominator. To rename $\dfrac{1}{3}$, multiply the numerator and the denominator by 3.

$$\frac{1 \times 3}{3 \times 3} = \frac{3}{9}$$

3. Because the denominator of the second fraction is 9, no change is necessary.
4. Add the numerators together, and keep the common denominator.
5. Reduce the fraction if necessary.

Addition of Mixed Numbers

Example

$$2\frac{1}{3} + 3\frac{11}{15}$$

$$2\frac{1 \times 5}{3 \times 5} = 2\frac{5}{15}$$

$$3\frac{11 \times 1}{15 \times 1} = 3\frac{11}{15}$$

$$2\frac{5}{15} + 3\frac{11}{15} = 5\frac{16}{15} = 6\frac{1}{15}$$

Steps

1. Find the LCD of 3 and 15 by listing the multiples of each.
   - 3 (3, 6, 9, 12, **15**)
   - 15 (**15**, 30, 45)
2. Calculate the new numerator of each fraction to correspond to the common denominator.
3. Add the whole numbers together, and then add the numerators together. Keep the common denominator 15.
4. The numerator is larger than the denominator (improper); change the answer to a mixed number (review vocabulary if necessary).

SAMPLE PROBLEMS

Add the fractions in the following problems as indicated (reduce fractions to lowest terms and change improper fractions to mixed numbers).

1. $\dfrac{2}{4} + \dfrac{1}{4} =$

2. $\dfrac{3}{21} + \dfrac{7}{21} =$

3. $\dfrac{4}{6} + \dfrac{7}{6} =$

4. $\dfrac{5}{8} + \dfrac{1}{16} =$

5. $\dfrac{7}{9} + \dfrac{6}{11} =$

6. $6\dfrac{2}{3} + 4\dfrac{5}{12} =$

7. $2\dfrac{2}{7} + 3\dfrac{2}{9} =$

8. $5\dfrac{1}{6} + 3\dfrac{2}{18} =$

9. Ray is driving Tom to the movies. Tom lives $2\frac{1}{2}$ miles from Ray's house. The movie theatre is $1\frac{3}{4}$ miles from Tom's house. How many miles must Ray drive to pick up Tom and drive to the theatre?

10. The Warrens are installing a privacy fence along two sides of their property. The length of one side is $85\frac{1}{3}$ feet. The length of the other side is $62\frac{5}{6}$ feet. How many feet of fencing will the Warrens install?

Subtraction of Fractions

Subtracting Fractions with Common Denominators

Example

$$\frac{5}{6} - \frac{1}{6} = \frac{4}{6} = \frac{2}{3}$$

Steps

1. Subtract the numerators: (5 − 1 = 4)
2. Keep the common denominator.
3. Reduce the fraction by dividing by the greatest common factor:

$$\frac{4}{6} \div \frac{2}{2} = \frac{2}{3}$$

Subtracting Fractions with Unlike Denominators

Example

$$\frac{5}{12} - \frac{1}{8} = ?$$

$$\frac{5 \times 2}{12 \times 2} = \frac{10}{24}$$

$$\frac{1 \times 3}{8 \times 3} = \frac{3}{24}$$

$$\frac{10}{24} - \frac{3}{24} = \frac{7}{24}$$

Steps

1. Find the LCD by listing the multiples of each denominator.
   - 12 {12, **24**, 36, 48}
   - 8 {8, 16, **24**, 32}
   - The LCD is 24.
2. Change the numerator to reflect the new denominator. (What is done to the bottom must be done to the top of a fraction.)
3. Subtract the new numerators: $10 - 3 = 7$. The denominator stays the same.

Borrowing from Whole Numbers

Example

$$4\frac{2}{3} - 3\frac{5}{7}$$

$$4\frac{2 \times 7}{3 \times 7} = 4\frac{14}{21}$$

$$^{3}\cancel{4}\frac{14}{21} + \frac{21}{21} = 3\frac{35}{21}$$

$$3\frac{5 \times 3}{7 \times 3} = 3\frac{15}{21}$$

$$3\frac{35}{21} - 3\frac{15}{21} = \frac{20}{21}$$

Steps

1. Find the LCD.
2. Fifteen cannot be subtracted from 14; therefore, 1 must be borrowed from the whole number, making it 3, and the borrowed 1 must be added to the fraction.
3. Add the original numerator to the borrowed numerator: $14 + 21 = 35$.
4. Now the whole number and the numerator can be subtracted.

SAMPLE PROBLEMS

Subtract the fractions in the following problems as indicated. (If necessary, convert improper fractions to mixed numbers.)

1. $\dfrac{4}{5} - \dfrac{2}{5} =$

2. $\dfrac{19}{21} - \dfrac{8}{21} =$

3. $\dfrac{2}{4} - \dfrac{3}{16} =$

4. $\dfrac{27}{56} - \dfrac{3}{7} =$

5. $1\dfrac{2}{5} - \dfrac{1}{2} =$

6. $16\dfrac{8}{9} - 5\dfrac{2}{3} =$

7. $11\dfrac{1}{5} - 8\dfrac{4}{5} =$

8. $20\dfrac{1}{2} - 4\dfrac{2}{3} =$

9. Terry has $8\frac{1}{4}$ feet of wood trim. He needs $5\frac{1}{3}$ feet of trim to decorate one wall. After cutting the wood to size, how much trim will Terry have left?

10. Jordan has a gallon of milk, which is equal to 16 cups. She uses $1\frac{1}{4}$ cups of milk to make pancakes. How many cups of milk does Jordan have left after making pancakes?

Multiplication of Fractions

Example 1

$$\frac{2}{3} \times \frac{5}{8}$$

$$\frac{2}{3} \times \frac{5}{8} = \frac{10}{24} = \frac{5}{12}$$

Steps

1. Multiply the numerators together: $2 \times 5 = 10$.
2. Multiply the denominators together: $3 \times 8 = 24$.
3. Reduce the product by using the greatest common factor: $\frac{10 \div 2}{24 \div 2} = \frac{5}{12}$

Example 2

$$5 \times \frac{4}{13}$$

$$\frac{5}{1} \times \frac{4}{13} = \frac{20}{13} = 1\frac{7}{13}$$

Steps

1. Make the whole number 5 into a fraction by placing a 1 as the denominator.
2. Multiply the numerators: $5 \times 4 = 20$.
3. Multiply the denominators: $1 \times 13 = 13$.
4. Change the improper fraction into a mixed number.

Example 3

$$3\frac{1}{6} \times 6\frac{5}{8}$$

$$\frac{19}{6} \times \frac{53}{8} = \frac{1,007}{48}$$

$$\frac{1,007}{48} = 20\frac{47}{48}$$

Steps

1. Change the mixed numbers into improper fractions.

$$3\frac{+1}{\times 6} = (3 \times 6) + 1 = 19 \rightarrow \frac{19}{6}$$

$$6\frac{+5}{\times 8} = (6 \times 8) + 5 = 53 \rightarrow \frac{53}{8}$$

2. Multiply the numerators and denominators together.
   - $19 \times 53 = 1,007$ (numerator)
   - $6 \times 8 = 48$ (denominator)
   - Change the improper fraction into a mixed number.

$$48\overline{)1007} = 20\frac{47}{48}$$
$$\underline{-96}$$
$$47$$
with quotient 20 above.

Multiply the following fractions (reduce the product to lowest terms and change improper fractions to mixed numbers).

1. $\dfrac{4}{7} \times \dfrac{1}{4} =$

2. $\dfrac{5}{7} \times \dfrac{2}{3} =$

3. $5 \times \dfrac{7}{6} =$

4. $2\dfrac{6}{7} \times 7 =$

5. $5\dfrac{5}{8} \times 2\dfrac{5}{6} =$

6. $3\dfrac{1}{6} \times 1\dfrac{4}{5} =$

7. $2\dfrac{3}{4} \times 3 =$

8. $1\dfrac{3}{9} \times 3\dfrac{1}{4} =$

9. A baseball pitcher throws an average of 15 pitches per inning. This pitcher throws an average of $6\frac{1}{3}$ innings per game. What is the average number of pitches per game for this pitcher?

10. Kelly's smartphone has a battery life of $10\frac{1}{6}$ hours. She buys a new phone with a battery life that is $1\frac{1}{2}$ times longer than her current phone. How many hours of battery life does her new phone have?

Division of Fractions

HESI Hint

"Dividing fractions, don't ask why, inverse the second fraction and then multiply."

Example:

$$\dfrac{1}{2} \div \dfrac{3}{8} \text{ Inverse } \dfrac{3}{8} \rightarrow \dfrac{8}{3}$$

$$\text{Then multiply } \dfrac{1}{2} \times \dfrac{8}{3}$$

$$\dfrac{1}{2} \times \dfrac{8}{3} = \dfrac{8}{6}$$

Write as a mixed number: $1\dfrac{2}{6}$ then reduce to lowest terms: $1\dfrac{1}{3}$

$$\dfrac{3}{8} \rightarrow \dfrac{8}{3} \quad \dfrac{3}{8} \times \dfrac{8}{3} = \dfrac{24}{24} = 1$$

These two numbers $\left(\dfrac{3}{8} \text{ and } \dfrac{8}{3}\right)$ are **reciprocals** of each other because they equal 1 when they are multiplied together.

Example 1

$$\dfrac{1}{3} \div \dfrac{3}{4}$$

$$\frac{1}{3} \div \frac{3}{4}$$

$$\frac{1}{3} \times \frac{4}{3} = \frac{4}{9}$$

Steps

1. Invert (or take the reciprocal of) the second fraction: $\frac{3}{4} \to \frac{4}{3}$.

2. Rewrite the new problem and multiply.
   - $1 \times 4 = 4$ (numerator)
   - $3 \times 3 = 9$ (denominator)

Example 2

$$1\frac{5}{6} \div \frac{3}{4}$$

$$1\frac{5}{6} \div \frac{3}{4}$$

$$\frac{11}{6} \div \frac{3}{4}$$

$$\frac{11}{6} \times \frac{4}{3} = \frac{44}{18}$$

$$2\frac{8}{18} = 2\frac{4}{9}$$

Steps

1. Change the mixed number to an improper fraction: $1\frac{5}{6} = (1 \times 6) + 5 = \frac{11}{6}$.

2. Rewrite the new problem with the improper fraction.
3. Invert the second fraction.
4. Multiply the numerators and the denominators together.
   - $11 \times 4 = 44$ (numerators)
   - $6 \times 3 = 18$ (denominators)
5. Change the improper fraction to a mixed number. Reduce the mixed number.

Example 3

$$9 \div 3\frac{2}{3}$$

$$\frac{9}{1} \div \frac{11}{3}$$

$$\frac{9}{1} \times \frac{3}{11} = \frac{27}{11}$$

$$2\frac{5}{11}$$

Steps

1. Change the whole number to a fraction and the mixed number to an improper fraction.
2. Invert the second fraction.
3. Multiply the numerators and the denominators together.
   - $9 \times 3 = 27$
   - $1 \times 11 = 11$
4. Change the improper fraction to a mixed number.

SAMPLE PROBLEMS

Divide the fractions and reduce to the lowest terms.

1. $\dfrac{5}{6} \div \dfrac{1}{6} =$

2. $\dfrac{4}{7} \div \dfrac{1}{4} =$

3. $\dfrac{3}{8} \div \dfrac{2}{6} =$

4. $2 \div \dfrac{1}{7} =$

5. $6 \div \dfrac{2}{5} =$

6. $6\dfrac{2}{3} \div \dfrac{1}{3} =$

7. $7 \div 2\dfrac{1}{3} =$

8. $16\dfrac{2}{5} \div 4 =$

9. Gary has 1½ pounds of chicken. A recipe for chicken tacos allows for ⅛ pounds of chicken for each taco. How many tacos can Gary make?

10. Patty makes decorative wreaths. She has 31¼ feet of ribbon to make bows for her wreaths. Each bow requires 6¼ feet of ribbon. How many wreaths can Patty make?

Changing Fractions to Decimals

HESI Hint

"Top goes in the box, the bottom goes out."

This is a helpful saying in remembering that the numerator is the dividend and the denominator is the divisor.

If the decimal does not terminate, continue to the thousandths place and then round to the hundredths place.

Example:

7.8666 → 7.87

If the number in the thousandths place is 5 or greater, round the number in the hundredths place to the next higher number. However, if the number in the thousandths place is less than 5, do not round up the number in the hundredths place.

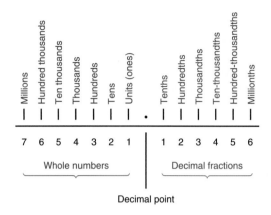

Millions	Hundred thousands	Ten thousands	Thousands	Hundreds	Tens	Units (ones)		Tenths	Hundredths	Thousandths	Ten-thousandths	Hundred-thousandths	Millionths

$$7 \quad 6 \quad 5 \quad 4 \quad 3 \quad 2 \quad 1 \quad\Big|\quad 1 \quad 2 \quad 3 \quad 4 \quad 5 \quad 6$$

Whole numbers   Decimal fractions

Decimal point

Example 1

Change $\dfrac{1}{4}$ to a decimal.

$$
\begin{array}{r}
0.25 \\
4\overline{)1.00} \\
-8\downarrow \\
\hline
20 \\
-20 \\
\hline
0
\end{array}
$$

Steps

1. Change the fraction into a division problem.
2. Add a decimal point after the 1 and add two zeros.
   - Remember to raise the decimal into the quotient area.
3. The answer is a **terminating decimal** (a decimal that is not continuous); therefore, adding additional zeros is not necessary.

Example 2

Change $\dfrac{5}{8}$ to a decimal.

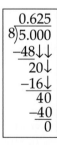

$$
\begin{array}{r}
0.625 \\
8\overline{)5.000} \\
-48\downarrow\downarrow \\
\hline
20\downarrow \\
-16\downarrow \\
\hline
40 \\
-40 \\
\hline
0
\end{array}
$$

Steps

1. Change the fraction into a division problem.
2. Add a decimal point after the 5 and add two zeros.
   - Remember to raise the decimal into the quotient area.
3. If there is still a remainder, add another zero to the dividend and bring it down.
4. The decimal terminates at the thousandths place.

Example 3

Change $\frac{1}{6}$ to a decimal.

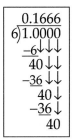

Steps

1. Change the fraction into a division problem.
2. After the 1, add a decimal point and two zeros.
3. The decimal continues (does not terminate); therefore, round to the hundredths place: 0.1666 → 0.167. (It can also be written as $0.1\overline{6}$. The line is placed over the number that repeats.)

Example 4

Change $3\frac{3}{4}$ to a decimal.

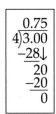

Steps

1. Change the fraction into a division problem.
2. After the 3, add a decimal and two zeros.
3. Place the whole number in front of the decimal: 3.75.

SAMPLE PROBLEMS

Change the following fractions into decimals. (If rounding is necessary, round to the nearest hundredth.)

1. $\frac{1}{7}$

2. $\frac{3}{11}$

3. $\frac{5}{8}$

4. $\frac{2}{4}$

5. $\frac{2}{5}$

6. $1\frac{1}{4}$

7. $\frac{3}{12}$

8. $3\frac{3}{5}$

9. $9\frac{3}{16}$

10. $\frac{17}{25}$

Changing Decimals to Fractions

Example 1

Change 0.9 to a fraction.

$$0.9 \rightarrow \frac{9}{10}$$

Steps

Knowing place values makes it very simple to change decimals to fractions.
1. The last digit is located in the tenths place; therefore, the 9 becomes the numerator.
2. 10 becomes the denominator.

Example 2

Change 0.02 to a fraction.

$$0.02 \rightarrow \frac{2}{100} = \frac{1}{50}$$

Steps

1. The 2 is located in the hundredths place.
2. The numerator becomes 2, and 100 becomes the denominator.
3. Reduce the fraction.

Example 3

Change 0.75 to a fraction.

$$0.75 \rightarrow \frac{75}{100} = \frac{3}{4}$$

Steps

1. Always look at the last digit in the decimal. In this example, the 5 is located in the hundredths place.

2. The numerator becomes 75, and 100 becomes the denominator.
3. Reduce the fraction.

Change 2.045 into a fraction.

$$2.045 \rightarrow 2\frac{45}{1000} \rightarrow 2\frac{9}{200}$$

Steps

1. The 5 is located in the thousandths place.
2. The numerator becomes 45, and 1000 becomes the denominator. The 2 is still the whole number.
3. Reduce the fraction.

SAMPLE PROBLEMS

Change the following decimals into fractions and reduce to the lowest terms.
1. 0.11 =
2. 0.25 =
3. 0.175 =
4. 0.22 =
5. 0.8 =
6. 4.25 =
7. 6.4 =
8. 10.6667 =
9. 8.24 =
10. 0.075 =

Ratios and Proportions

Ratio: A relationship between two numbers.
Proportion: Two ratios that have equal values.

HESI Hint

Ratios can be written several ways.
As a fraction: $\frac{5}{12}$
Using a colon: 5:12
In words: 5 to 12
Proportions can be written two ways.

$$\frac{5}{12} = \frac{25}{60}$$
$$5:12::25:60$$

NOTE: The numerator is listed first, then the denominator.

Example 1

Change the decimal to a ratio.

$$0.012 \rightarrow \frac{12}{1000} \rightarrow \frac{3}{250} \rightarrow 3:250$$

Steps

1. Change the decimal to a fraction.
2. Reduce the fraction.
3. The numerator (3) is the first listed number.
4. Then write the colon.
5. Finally, place the denominator (250) after the colon.

Example 2

Change the fraction to a ratio.

$$\frac{4}{5} = 4:5$$

Steps

1. The numerator (4) is the first listed number.
2. Then write the colon.
3. Finally, place the denominator (5) after the colon.

Example 3

Solve the proportion (find the value of x).

$2:7 : : 8{:}x$

$$2{:}7 :: 8{:}x$$
$$\frac{2}{7} = \frac{8}{x}$$
$$\frac{2}{7} = \frac{8}{x}$$
$$\frac{2}{7} = \frac{8}{x}$$
$$x = 28$$

Steps

1. Rewrite the proportion as a fraction.
2. Cross-multiply (multiply diagonally):
   - $2 \times x = 2x$
   - $7 \times 8 = 56$
3. Solve for x:
   - $2x = 56$ (divide both sides by 2)
   - $x = 28$

Example 4

Solve the proportion (find the value of x).

$x{:}28 : : 12{:}48$

$$\frac{x}{28} = \frac{12}{48}$$

$$\frac{x}{28} = \frac{12}{48}$$

$$12 \times 28 = 336$$
$$336 \div 48 = 7$$
$$x = 7$$

Steps

1. Rewrite the proportion as a fraction.
2. Cross-multiply:
   - $x \times 48 = 48x$
   - $28 \times 12 = 336$.
3. Solve for x:
   - $48x = 336$ (divide both sides by 48)
   - $x = 7$

Example 5

Solve the proportion (find the value of x).
   240:60 : : x:12.

$$\frac{240}{60} = \frac{x}{12}$$

$$\frac{240}{60} = \frac{x}{12}$$

$$x = 48$$

Steps

1. Rewrite the proportion as a fraction.
2. Cross-multiply:
   - $240 \times 12 = 2,880$
   - $60 \times x = 60x$
3. Solve for x:
   - $60x = 2,880$ (divide both sides by 60)
   - $x = 48$

SAMPLE PROBLEMS

Change the following fractions to ratios.

1. $\dfrac{12}{43}$

2. $\dfrac{7}{30}$

Solve the following for x:

3. 4:5 : : 28:x

4. 15:4 : : x:16

5. x:12 : : 29:116
6. 27:x : : 9:13
7. 126:72 : : 14:x
8. x:144 : : 12:36
9. If Barb types 130 words in 2 minutes, how long will it take her to type 325 words?
10. Steve is a painter. He needs 25 gallons of paint to cover 10 offices. Assuming all the offices are the same size, how many gallons of paint does Steve need to finish painting 3 offices?

Percentages

Percent: Per hundred (part per hundred).

Example 1

Change the decimal to a **percent:** 0.31 → 31%.

Steps

1. Move the decimal point to the right of the hundredths place (two places).
2. Put the percent sign behind the new number.

Example 2

Change the decimal to a percent: 0.007 → 0.7%.

Steps

1. Move the decimal point to the right of the hundredths place (always two places!).
2. Put the percent sign behind the new number.

Example 3

Change the percent to a decimal: 73.2% → 0.732.

Steps

1. Move the decimal two spaces away from the percent sign (to the left).
2. Drop the percent sign; it is no longer a percent, but a decimal.

Example 4

Change the percent to a decimal: 25% → 0.25.

Steps

1. The decimal point is not visible, but is always located after the last number.
2. Move the decimal two spaces away from the percent sign (toward the left).
3. Drop the percent sign; the number is no longer a percent, but a decimal.

Example 5

Change the fraction to a percent: $\dfrac{8}{9}$

$$
\begin{array}{r}
.888 \\
9\overline{)8.000} \\
-72\downarrow\downarrow \\
\hline
80\downarrow \\
-72\downarrow \\
\hline
80
\end{array}
$$

$0.888 \rightarrow 88.8\%$

Steps

1. Change the fraction into a division problem and solve.
2. Move the decimal behind the hundredths place in the quotient.
3. Place a percent sign after the new number.

SAMPLE PROBLEMS

Change the following decimals to percents.
1. $0.99 =$
2. $0.027 =$
3. $0.0052 =$
   Change the following percents to decimals.
4. $1.1\% =$
5. $8\% =$
6. $0.9\% =$
   Change the following fractions to percents (if rounding is necessary, round to the nearest tenths place).
7. $\dfrac{7}{10} =$
8. $\dfrac{2}{5} =$
9. $\dfrac{5}{6} =$
10. $\dfrac{1}{8} =$

Using the Percent Formula

HESI Hint

The word *of* usually indicates the whole portion of the percent formula.
Percent formula:

$$\frac{\text{Part}}{\text{Whole}} = \frac{\%}{100}$$

Using this formula will help in all percent problems in which there is an unknown (solving for *x*).

Example 1

What is 7 out of 8 expressed as a percent?

$$\frac{7}{8} = \frac{\%}{100}$$

$$7 \times 100 = 700$$
$$700 \div 8 = 87.5$$
$$\% = 87.5 \text{ or } 87.5\%$$

Steps

1. Rewrite the problem using the percent formula.
2. Multiply the diagonal numbers together: $7 \times 100 = 700$.
3. Divide by the remaining number: $700 \div 8 = 87.5\%$.

Example 2

What is 32% of 75?

$$\frac{x}{75} = \frac{32}{100}$$

$$75 \times 32 = 2{,}400$$
$$2{,}400 \div 100 = 24$$
$$x = 24$$

Steps

1. Rewrite the problem using the percent formula.
2. "Of 75:" 75 is the whole.
3. Multiply the diagonal numbers together: $75 \times 32 = 2{,}400$.
4. Divide by the remaining number: $2{,}400 \div 100 = 24$.
5. $x = 24$ (this is not a percent; it is the part).

Example 3

14 is 56% of what number?

$$\frac{14}{x} = \frac{56}{100}$$

$$14 \times 100 = 1{,}400$$
$$1{,}400 \div 56 = 25$$
$$x = 25$$

Steps

1. Rewrite the problem using the percent formula.
2. We are looking for the **whole** because *of* is indicating an unknown number.
3. Multiply the diagonal numbers together: $14 \times 100 = 1{,}400$.
4. Divide by the remaining number: $1{,}400 \div 56 = 25$.

Fractions, Decimals, and Percents

Fraction	Decimal	Percent
$\frac{1}{2}$	0.50	50%
$\frac{1}{4}$	0.25	25%
$\frac{3}{4}$	0.75	75%
$\frac{1}{5}$	0.20	20%
$\frac{2}{5}$	0.40	40%
$\frac{3}{5}$	0.60	60%
$\frac{4}{5}$	0.80	80%
$\frac{1}{8}$	0.125	12.5%
$\frac{3}{8}$	0.375	37.5%
$\frac{5}{8}$	0.625	62.5%
$\frac{7}{8}$	0.875	87.5%
$\frac{1}{3}$	0.333	33.3%
$\frac{2}{3}$	0.666	66.6%

SAMPLE PROBLEMS

Solve the following percent problems
1. What is 14 out of 56 as a percent?
2. What is 2 out of 80 as a percent?
3. What is 45 out of 150 as a percent?
4. What is 75% of 32?
5. What is 65% of 40?
6. What is 2.5% of 400?
7. The number 5 is 20% of what number?
8. The number 30 is 25% of what number?
9. The number 9 is 30% of what number?
10. The number 51 is 25% of what number?

Mean, Median, and Mode

Mean, median, and mode are measures that describe a center, or a central tendency, within a set of data points.

Mean: The sum of all the values in a data set divided by the number of values; often called the *average.*

Median: The middle number of a data set arranged in numerical order.

Mode: The number that appears most often in a data set.

Example 1

Find the mean for the following set of values:

1, 3, 3, 9, 7, 8, 4

Steps

1. Calculate the sum of the values:
   $1 + 3 + 3 + 9 + 7 + 8 + 4 = 35$
2. Divide by the number of values:
   $35 \div 7 =$
3. Answer: 5

Example 2

Find the median for the following set of values:

6, 7, 7, 2, 9, 5, 3, 1

Steps

1. Arrange the values in numerical order:
   1, 2, 3, 5, 6, 7, 7, 9
2. Find the middle number (when there is an even amount of numbers, add the two middle numbers):
   1, 2, 3, 5, 6, 7, 7, 9
   $5 + 6 = 11$
3. Divide by 2:
   $11 \div 2 =$
4. Answer: 5.5

Example 3

Find the mode for the following set of values:

4, 7, 9, 9, 10, 12, 15

Steps

1. Find the value that appears most often:
   4, 7, 9, 9, 10, 12, 15
2. Answer: 9

SAMPLE PROBLEMS

Find the mean, median, and mode for the following set of numbers:

3, 12, 3, 25, 34, 1, 0, 1, 3

1. Mean: _____
2. Median: _____
3. Mode: _____

Find the mean, median, and mode for the following set of numbers:
13, 17, 11, 21, 11, 14, 8, 19
4. Mean: _____
5. Median: _____
6. Mode: _____
   Find the mean and median for the following set of numbers:
   4, 6, 7, 8, 9, 10, 19
7. Mean: _____
8. Median: _____
   Find the mean and median for the following set of numbers:
   2, 12, 6, 21, 5, 8, 3, 11
9. Mean: _____
10. Median: _____

Algebra

Variable: A letter representing an unknown quantity (i.e., x).
Constant: A number that cannot change.
Expression: A mathematical sentence containing constants and variables (i.e., $3x - 2$).
Exponent: A raised number or symbol (i.e., a superscript) placed after another number or symbol, indicating the number of times to multiply.

Algebra is a process that involves variables and constants. A **variable** is a letter that represents an unknown quantity. A **constant** is a number that cannot change. Using the operations of addition, subtraction, multiplication, and division, we can use algebra to determine the value of unknown quantities. Two algebra concepts discussed in this section will be evaluating **expressions** and solving equations for a specific variable.

HESI Hint

When working with algebra, remember to evaluate expressions by performing the "Order of Operations."

Order of Operations
1. Evaluate numbers within parentheses. $4 \cdot (2+3)^2 - 5$
2. Multiply numbers based on any exponents. $4 \cdot (5)^2 - 5$
3. Multiply and divide numbers from left to right. $4 \cdot 25 - 5$
4. Add and subtract numbers from left to right. $4 \cdot 25 - 5$
   Here's a mnemonic to remember the "Order of Operations":
   "Please excuse my dear Aunt Sally" helps to remember the correct order of operations.
   The order should be Parentheses, Exponents, Multiply, Divide, Add, Subtract.

Evaluating the Expression

- Numbers can be positive (1 or +1) or negative (-1). If a number has no sign (e.g., 1) it usually means it is a positive number.
- Adding positive numbers is similar to addition (e.g., $1 + 3 = 4$).
- Subtracting positive numbers is simple subtraction (e.g., $4 - 3 = 1$).
- Subtracting a negative number is the same as adding (e.g., $3 - [-1] = 4$); it is written as $3 + 1 = 4$.

- Subtracting a positive number: $4 - (+3) = 4 - 3 = 1$
- Adding a negative number: $3 + (-4) = 3 - 4 = -1$

Rules

- Two like signs become positive signs: $3 + (+1) = 3 + 1 = 4$

$$3 - (-1) = 3 + 1 = 4$$

- Two unlike signs become a negative sign: $8 + (-2) = 8 - 2 = 6$

$$8 - (+2) = 8 - 2 = 6$$

When we substitute a specific value for each variable in the expression and then perform the operations, it's called "evaluating the expression."

Example 1

Evaluate the expression $ab + c$ if $a = 6$, $b = -4$, and $c = 12$

$$(6)(-4) + 12$$
$$-24 + 12$$
$$-12$$

Steps

1. Substitute the numbers into the given expression. Use parentheses when inserting numbers into an expression.
2. Multiply $6 \times -4 = -24$
3. Add $-24 + 12 = -12$

Example 2

Evaluate the expression $-xy(x - y) + y$ if $x = 5$ and $y = -1$
$$-(5)(-1)([5] - [-1]) + (-1)$$
$$-(-5)(5 + 1) - 1$$
$$5(6) - 1$$
$$30 - 1$$
$$29$$

Steps

1. Substitute the numbers into the given expression:
   - $-(5)(-1)([5] - [-1]) + (-1)$
2. Solve operations inside parentheses:
   - $[5] - [-1] = 6$
3. Rewrite expression:
   - $-(5)(-1)(6) + (-1)$
4. Multiply from left to right:
   - $-(5)(-1) = 5$
   - $(5)(6) = 30$
5. Add/subtract:
   - $30 + (-1)$
   - $30 - 1 = 29$

Solving Equations for a Specific Variable

To solve equations for a specific variable, perform the operations in the reverse order in which you evaluate expressions.

Example 3

Solve: $2x + 3 = 21$

$$\frac{\overset{-3}{2x}}{2} = \frac{\overset{-3}{18}}{2}$$

$$x = 9$$

Steps

Isolate the variable by subtracting 3 from both sides of the equation:
- $2x + 3 - 3 = 21 - 3$
- $2x = 18$

2. Divide both sides by 2:
- $\dfrac{2x}{2} = \dfrac{18}{2}$

3. Solve:
- $x = 9$

Example 4

Solve: $-4k - 2 = -17$

$$\frac{\overset{+2}{-4k}}{-4} = \frac{\overset{+2}{-15}}{-4}$$

$$k = \frac{15}{4}$$

Steps

1. Add 2 to both sides.
2. Divide both sides by −4.
3. Simplify. (A negative divided by a negative is a positive.)

SAMPLE PROBLEMS

Evaluate the following expressions:
1. $x + 9y$ if $x = 3$ and $y = -2$
2. $2ab - am$ if $a = 1$, $b = 2$, and $m = -2$
3. $-2x(y - 2z)$ if $x = 3$, $y = -2$, and $z = 6$
4. $-qr + r - s$ if $q = 2$, $r = 4$, and $s = 6$
5. $(a + b)(2a + bc)$ if $a = 4$, $b = -2$, and $c = 3$

Solve the following equations for the given variable:
6. $6x - 6 = 24$ solve for x.
7. $-x - 4 = 18$ solve for x.
8. $4y + 15 = 28$ solve for y.
9. $4x - 12 = -4$ solve for x.
10. $-5 = 8a + 3$ solve for a.

Other Helpful Information

Equivalents for Military Time and 12-hour Clock Time

Military Time	12-hour Clock Time	Military Time	12-hour Clock Time
0000	12:00 AM (Midnight)	1200	12:00 PM (Noon)
0100	1:00 AM	1300	1:00 PM
0200	2:00 AM	1400	2:00 PM
0300	3:00 AM	1500	3:00 PM
0400	4:00 AM	1600	4:00 PM
0500	5:00 AM	1700	5:00 PM
0600	6:00 AM	1800	6:00 PM
0700	7:00 AM	1900	7:00 PM
0800	8:00 AM	2000	8:00 PM
0900	9:00 AM	2100	9:00 PM
1000	10:00 AM	2200	10:00 PM
1100	11:00 AM	2300	11:00 PM

HESI Hint

To convert to military time before noon, simply include a zero before the numbers 1 through 9 for AM. For example, 9:35 AM 12-hour clock time converts to 0935 military time. The zero is not needed when converting 10 AM or 11 AM. If the time is after noon, simply add 12 to the hour number. For example, 1:30 PM 12-hour clock time converts to 1330 military time ($1 + 12 = 13$). Midnight, or 12 AM, is converted to 0000. Noon, or 12 PM, is converted to 1200.

Roman Numerals

I = 1	XX = 20	M = 1,000
II = 2	XXX = 30	V = 5,000
III = 3	XL = 40	X = 10,000
IV = 4	L = 50	L = 50,000
V = 5	LX = 60	C = 100,000
VI = 6	LXX = 70	D = 500,000
VII = 7	LXXX = 80	M = 1,000,000
VIII = 8	XC = 90	
IX = 9	C = 100	
X = 10	D = 500	
XI = 11		
Example 2012 = MMXII		

Measurement Conversions

Temperature
0° Celsius = 32° Fahrenheit (the freezing point of water)
Celsius to Fahrenheit
The temperature T in degrees Fahrenheit (°F) is equal to the temperature T in degrees Celsius (°C) times $\frac{9}{5}$ plus 32: $T_{(°F)} = T_{(°C)} \times 9/5 + 32$ or $T_{(°F)} = T_{(°C)} \times 1.8 + 32$ **Example** $T_{(°F)} = 20°C \times \frac{9}{5} + 32 = 68°F$
100° Celsius = 212° Fahrenheit (the boiling point of water)
Fahrenheit to Celsius
0 degrees Fahrenheit is equal to −17.77778 degrees Celsius: $0°F = −17.77778°C$ The temperature T in degrees Celsius (°C) is equal to the temperature T in degrees Fahrenheit (°F) minus 32, times $\frac{5}{9}$: $T_{(°C)} = (T_{(°F)} − 32) \times \frac{5}{9}$ or $T_{(°C)} = (T_{(°F)} − 32) \div \left(\frac{9}{5}\right)$ or $T_{(°C)} = (T_{(°F)} − 32) \div 1.8$ **Example** Convert 68 degrees Fahrenheit to degrees Celsius: $T_{(°C)} = (68°F − 32) \times \frac{5}{9} = 20°C$

Length

Metric	*English*
1 kilometer = 1,000 meters	1 mile = 1,760 yards
1 meter = 100 centimeters	1 mile = 5,280 feet
1 centimeter = 10 millimeters	1 yard = 3 feet
2.54 centimeters = 1 inch	1 foot = 12 inches

Volume and Capacity

Metric	*English*
1 liter = 1,000 milliliters	1 gallon = 4 quarts
1 milliliter = 1 cubic centimeter	1 gallon = 128 ounces
	1 quart = 2 pints
	1 pint = 2 cups
	1 cup = 8 ounces
	1 ounce = 30 milliliters (cubic centimeters)

Weight and Mass

Metric	*English*
1 kilogram = 1,000 grams	1 ton = 2,000 pounds
1 gram = 1,000 milligrams	1 pound = 16 ounces
	2.2 pounds = 1 kilogram

ANSWERS TO SAMPLE PROBLEMS

Basic Addition and Subtraction
1. 2,043
2. 320
3. 2,001
4. 306
5. 232
6. 199
7. 6,122
8. 16,521
9. 7
10. 9

Basic Multiplication (Whole Numbers)
1. 2,052
2. 4,599
3. 18,062
4. 24,863
5. 71,550
6. 24,628
7. 65,067
8. 862,299
9. 1,656
10. 676

Basic Division (Whole Numbers)
1. 12.75
2. 800
3. 1,866
4. 21
5. 525
6. 975
7. 98.375
8. 1,256.2
9. 4.5
10. 15

Addition and Subtraction of Decimals
1. 9.82
2. 50.445
3. 210.2
4. 52.57
5. 19.26
6. 7.82
7. 57.91
8. 7.68
9. 15.25
10. 1.75

Multiplication of Decimals
1. 4.077
2. 218.54
3. 24.644
4. 5,779.8
5. 7.408056
6. 148.4
7. 0.4068
8. 0.73572
9. 61.5
10. 4.8

Division of Decimals
1. 47
2. 293
3. 82
4. 62.2
5. 11.56
6. 4,560
7. 0.065
8. 2.4
9. 8
10. 4

Addition of Fractions
1. $\frac{3}{4}$
2. $\frac{10}{21}$
3. $1\frac{5}{6}$
4. $\frac{11}{16}$
5. $1\frac{32}{99}$
6. $11\frac{1}{12}$
7. $5\frac{32}{63}$
8. $8\frac{5}{18}$
9. $4\frac{1}{4}$
10. $148\frac{1}{6}$

Subtraction of Fractions

1. $\dfrac{2}{5}$

2. $\dfrac{11}{21}$

3. $\dfrac{5}{16}$

4. $\dfrac{3}{56}$

5. $\dfrac{9}{10}$

6. $11\dfrac{2}{9}$

7. $2\dfrac{2}{5}$

8. $15\dfrac{5}{6}$

9. $2\dfrac{11}{12}$

10. $14\dfrac{3}{4}$

Multiplication of Fractions

1. $\dfrac{1}{7}$

2. $\dfrac{10}{21}$

3. $5\dfrac{5}{6}$

4. 20

5. $15\dfrac{15}{16}$

6. $5\dfrac{7}{10}$

7. $8\dfrac{1}{4}$

8. $4\dfrac{1}{3}$

9. 95

10. $15\dfrac{1}{4}$

Division of Fractions

1. 5

2. 2 2/7

3. $1\dfrac{1}{8}$

4. 14

5. 15

6. 20

7. 3

8. $4\dfrac{1}{10}$

9. 12

10. 5

Changing Fractions to Decimals

1. 0.14

2. 0.27

3. 0.63

4. 0.5

5. 0.4

6. 1.25

7. 0.25

8. 3.6

9. 9.19

10. 0.68

Changing Decimals to Fractions

1. $\dfrac{11}{100}$

2. $\dfrac{1}{4}$

3. $\dfrac{7}{40}$

4. $\dfrac{11}{50}$

5. $\dfrac{4}{5}$

6. $4\dfrac{1}{4}$

7. $6\dfrac{2}{5}$

8. $10\dfrac{6667}{10000}$

9. $8\dfrac{6}{25}$

10. $\dfrac{3}{40}$

Ratios and Proportions

1. 12:43

2. 7:30

3. x = 35

4. x = 60

5. x = 3

6. x = 39

7. x = 8
8. x = 48
9. x = 5
10. x = 7.5

Percentages
1. 99%
2. 2.7%
3. 0.52%
4. 0.011
5. 0.08
6. 0.009
7. 70%
8. 40%
9. 83.3%
10. 12.5%

Using the Percent Formula
1. 25%
2. 2.5%
3. 30%
4. 24
5. 26
6. 10
7. 25
8. 120
9. 30
10. 204

Mean, Median, and Mode
1. 10
2. 3
3. 3
4. 14.25
5. 13.5
6. 11
7. 9
8. 8
9. 8.5
10. 7

Algebra
1. −15
2. 6
3. 84
4. −10
5. 4
6. x = 5
7. x = −22
8. $y = \dfrac{13}{4}$ or $y = 3\dfrac{1}{4}$
   or $y = 3.25$
9. x = 2
10. a = −1

READING COMPREHENSION

2

Information technology is constantly evolving and transforming the way we learn. Thanks to the Internet, we are able to communicate and share knowledge in ways that previous generations couldn't possibly imagine. Anyone with a computer, phone, or tablet can access virtually unlimited amounts of information with a mere click of a mouse or touch of a screen. However, our ability to benefit from this information depends entirely on our ability to understand it. This is why reading comprehension is an essential skill for students to develop. Comprehension is especially important in the healthcare setting, where accurate interpretation, recording, and sharing of information directly impacts patient care and outcomes. Patient assessment, diagnosis, treatment, care, progress, and outcome all depend on the ability of health professionals to understand what they read.

CHAPTER OUTLINE

KEY TERMS

Antonym
Assumption
Connotation

Context Clue
Inference
Purpose

Synonym
Tone

Identifying the Main Idea

Identifying the main idea is the key to understanding what has been read and what needs to be remembered. First, identify the topic of the passage or paragraph by asking the question, "What is it about?" Once that question has been answered, ask, "What point is the author making about the topic?" If the reader understands the author's message about the topic, the main idea has been identified.

In longer passages, the reader might find it helpful to count the number of paragraphs used to describe what is believed to be the main idea statement. If the majority of paragraphs include information about the main idea statement the reader has chosen, the reader is probably correct. However, if the answer chosen by the reader is mentioned in only one paragraph, the reader may have chosen a detail rather than the main idea.

Another helpful hint in identifying main ideas is to read a paragraph and then stop and summarize that paragraph. This type of active reading helps the reader focus on the content and can lessen the need to reread the entire passage several times.

Some students find that visualizing as they read helps them remember details and stay focused. Visualizing is a technique that helps students improve comprehension and recall by creating a picture of the information in their minds. (Think of visualization as making your own movie based on the information you read and projecting it onto a big-screen TV.) Informal classroom experiments have shown that students who use visualization techniques perform better on reading comprehension tests than their counterparts who do not visualize.

HESI Hint

Main ideas can be found in the beginning, in the middle, or at the end of a paragraph or passage. Always check the introduction and conclusion for the main idea of a passage.

Finally, not all main ideas are stated. Identify unstated or implied main ideas by looking specifically at the details, examples, causes, and reasons given.

Again, asking the questions stated earlier will help in this task:
- What is the passage about? (Topic)
- What point is the author making about the topic? (Main idea)

Some experts like to compare the main idea with an umbrella covering all or most of the details in a paragraph or passage. The chosen main idea can be tested for accuracy by asking whether the other details will fit under the umbrella. The idea of an umbrella also helps visualize how broad a statement the main idea can be.

Identifying Supporting Details

Writing comprises main ideas and details. Few individuals would enjoy reading only a writer's main ideas. The details provide the interest, the visual picture, and the examples that sustain a reader's interest.

Students often confuse the author's main idea with the examples or reasons the author gives to support the main idea. These details give the reader a description, the background, or simply more information to support the writer's assertion or main idea. Without these details, the reader would neither be able to evaluate whether the writer has made his or her case, nor would the reader find the passage as interesting. In addition to examples, facts and statistics may be used.

The reader's job is to distinguish the writer's main idea from details that support the main idea. Usually, the reader can discover clues to help identify details. For example, authors tend to use transition words such as *one, next, another, first,* or *finally* to indicate that a detail is being provided.

Finding the Meaning of Words in Context

Even the most avid readers will come across words that are unfamiliar to them. Identifying the correct meanings of these words may be the key to identifying the author's main idea and to fully comprehending the author's meaning. The reader can, of course, stop and use a dictionary or a thesaurus for these words. However, this is usually neither the most efficient nor the most practical way to approach unknown words.

There are other options the reader can use to find the meanings of unknown words, and these involve using context clues. The phrase **context clue** refers to the information provided by the author in the words or sentences surrounding the unknown word or words.

Some of the easiest context clues to recognize are as follows:

1. **Definition**—The author puts the meaning of the word in parentheses or states the definition in the following sentence.
2. **Synonym**—The author gives the reader another word that means the same or nearly the same as the unknown word.
3. **Antonym**—The author gives a word that means the opposite of the unknown word.

HESI Hint

The reader needs to watch for clue words such as *although*, *but*, and *instead*, which sometimes signal that an antonym is being used.

4. **Restatement**—The author restates the unknown word in a sentence using more familiar words.
5. **Examples**—The author gives examples that more clearly help the reader understand the meaning of the unknown word.
6. **Explanation**—The author gives more information about the unknown word, which better explains the meaning of the word.
7. **Word structure**—Sometimes simply knowing the meanings of basic prefixes, suffixes, and root words can help the reader make an educated guess about an unknown word.

HESI Hint

When being tested on finding the meaning of a word in the context of a passage, look carefully at the words and sentences surrounding the unknown word. The **context clues** are usually there for the reader to uncover. Once the correct meaning has been chosen, test that meaning in the passage. It should make sense, and the meaning should be supported by the other sentences in the passage or paragraph.

Identifying a Writer's Purpose and Tone

The purposes or reasons for reading or writing are similar for the readers and the writers. Readers read to be informed or entertained, and authors write to inform or entertain the reader. However, in the area of persuasion, a reader can be fooled into believing they are reading something objective when in fact the author is trying to influence or manipulate the reader's thinking, which is why it is important for readers to ask the following questions:

1. Who is the intended audience?
2. Why is this being written?

If the writer is trying to change the reader's thinking, encourage the reader to buy something, or convince the reader to vote for someone, the reader can assume the writer's goal is to persuade. More evidence can be found to determine the writer's purpose by identifying specific words used within the passage. Words that are biased, or words that have positive or negative connotations, will often help the reader determine the author's reason for writing. (**Connotation** refers to the emotions or feelings that the reader attaches to words.)

If the writer uses a number of words with negative or positive connotations, the writer is usually trying to influence the reader's thinking. Looking at the writer's choice of words also helps the reader determine the tone of the passage. (An author's **tone** refers to the attitude or feelings the author has about the topic.) Examples of tone in writing include formal, informal, entertaining, informative, light-hearted, tragic, positive (optimistic), and negative (pessimistic).

Identifying tone is especially important today, as we are constantly inundated with "breaking news" every time we turn on a TV or surf the Internet. If we pay close attention to the writer's choice of words and the types of details the writer chooses to include (or omit), we are better able to judge whether we are being informed or manipulated. For example, if a political writer states that a certain legislative proposal is "under attack" by "party radicals," the reader should be able to recognize that the writer is inserting personal bias and attempting to persuade the reader with provocative language. If another writer reports on the same topic using measured language while giving equal voice to both sides of the issue, it is likely that the writer is attempting to inform the reader.

Articles or books written to inform should be less biased, and information should be presented in factual format and with sufficient supporting data to allow readers to form their own opinions on the event that occurred.

HESI Hint

When determining the writer's purpose and/or tone, look closely at the writer's choice of words. The words are the key clues.

Distinguishing Between Fact and Opinion

A critical reader must be an active reader. A critical reader must question and evaluate the writer's underlying assumptions. An **assumption** is a set of beliefs that the writer has about the subject. A critical reader must determine whether the writer's statements are facts or opinions and whether the supporting evidence and details are relevant and valid. A critical reader is expected to determine whether the author's argument is credible and logical.

To distinguish between fact and opinion, the reader must understand the common definitions of those words. A fact is considered something that can be proved (either right or wrong). For example, at the time Columbus sailed for the New World, it was considered a scientific fact that the world was flat. Columbus proved the scientists wrong.

An opinion is a statement that cannot be proved. For example, "The movie *Boyhood* is the best movie ever made" is a statement of opinion. It is subjective; it is the writer's personal opinion. On the other hand, the following is a statement of fact: "The movie *Boyhood* was nominated for an Academy Award for best picture in 2015 but did not win." This statement is a fact because it can be proved to be correct.

Again, the reader must look closely at the writer's choice of words in determining the fact or opinion. Word choices that include measurable data and colors are considered factual or concrete words. "Frank weighs 220 pounds" and "Mary's dress is red" are examples of concrete words being used in statements of fact.

If the writer uses evaluative or judgmental words (*good, better, best, worst*), it is considered a statement of opinion. Abstract words (*love, hate, envy*) are also used in statements of opinion. These include ideas or concepts that cannot be measured. Statements that deal with probabilities or speculations about future events are also considered opinions.

Making Logical Inferences

In addition to determining fact and opinion, a critical reader is constantly required to make logical inferences. An **inference** is an educated guess or conclusion drawn by the reader based on the available facts and information. Although this may sound difficult and sometimes is, it is done frequently. A critical reader does not always know whether the inference is correct, but the inference is made based on the reader's own set of beliefs or assumptions.

Determining inferences is a skill often referred to as *reading between the lines*. It is a logical connection that is based on the situation, the facts provided, and the reader's knowledge and experience. The key to making logical inferences is to ensure that the inferences are supportable by evidence or facts presented in the reading. This often requires reading the passage twice so that details can be identified. Inferences are not stated in the reading but are derived from the information presented and influenced by the reader's knowledge and experience.

Summarizing

Identifying the best summary of a reading selection is a skill some students may find frustrating. Yet, this skill can be mastered easily when the following three rules are used:

1. The summary should include the main ideas from the beginning, middle, and end of the passage.
2. The summary is usually presented in sequence; however, occasionally it may be presented in a different order.
3. The summary must have accurate information. Sometimes a test summary will deliberately include false information. In that case, the critical reader will automatically throw out that test option.

Summary questions will typically take the longest for the student to answer because to answer them correctly, the student must go through each summary choice and locate the related information or main idea in the passage itself. Double-checking the summary choices is one way to verify that the reader has chosen the best summary. If the summary choice presents information that is inaccurate or out of order, the reader will automatically eliminate those choices.

HESI Hint

Remember, the summary should include the main ideas of the passage, possibly with some major supporting details. It is a shortened version of the passage that includes all the important information, eliminating the unnecessary and redundant.

REVIEW QUESTIONS

What makes some people do dangerous things? Most of us like to play it safe, and we instinctively avoid situations that pose a threat to our well-being. But some people thrive on danger and are driven by a need for intense excitement. Psychologists call these people "thrill-seekers." Thrill-seekers possess an irresistible urge to attempt dangerous feats with seemingly little regard for their own safety.

Notable examples of thrill-seeking include the many perilous attempts climbers have made to reach the summit of Mount Everest. The top portion of Everest is called the "death zone" because the extreme altitude and low atmospheric pressure make it difficult for climbers to breathe (or survive) for very long. Many people have died trying to reach the top of Everest, but many others still attempt the climb. The fascination some climbers have with conquering Everest is called "summit fever," which is marked by an intense desire to reach the top, despite certain and grave danger. Summit fever clouds the judgment of thrill-seeking climbers and prevents them from turning back, even when the chances of survival are bleak.

But what makes thrill-seekers different from the rest of us? Scientists say the answer may be related to the neurotransmitter dopamine. When a person perceives a dangerous situation, the brain releases dopamine, which produces the "high" a person feels after accomplishing a daring feat. But according to researchers, the thrill-seeker's brain has fewer dopamine-inhibiting receptors. This means their brains release more dopamine than normal during intense experiences, and as a result, they experience more intense highs. The dopamine high is so addictive that thrill-seekers are driven to take even greater risks as they keep chasing the next high.

Many of us may be tempted to dismiss thrill-seekers as "crazy" or "adrenaline junkies," but it would be a mistake to ridicule thrill-seekers without considering what our world might be like without them. Thrill-seekers have explored the ocean floor and blasted into outer space. They have navigated mysterious waters and discovered wonderous new lands. Without these intrepid souls, the human race may never have spread around the globe, built advanced civilizations, and developed the technologies that so many of us enjoy today.

1. What is the main idea of the second paragraph?
   - A. Thrill-seekers still attempt to climb Mount Everest despite the risks.
   - B. Attempting to climb Mount Everest is very dangerous.
   - C. Summit fever is an intense desire to reach the top of Mount Everest.
   - D. Mount Everest's high altitude makes it difficult to breathe.

2. Which response would be associated with high levels of dopamine in the brain?
   - A. Intense fear
   - B. Poor decision-making
   - C. Reduced stress
   - D. Increased pleasure

3. What is the meaning of the word *perilous* in the second paragraph?
   - A. Successful
   - B. Dangerous
   - C. Famous
   - D. Silly

4. What is the author's primary purpose in writing this essay?
   - A. To explain how neurotransmitters affect brain function
   - B. To explain why some people do dangerous things
   - C. To explain the consequences of thrill-seeking behavior
   - D. To explain why most people avoid dangerous situations

5. Identify the overall tone of the essay.
   - A. Negative
   - B. Tragic
   - C. Informative
   - D. Lighthearted

6. Which statement is an opinion expressed by the author?
   - A. Thrill-seekers are driven by a need for intense excitement.
   - B. Dopamine has been associated with thrill-seeking behavior.
   - C. The world might be better off because of thrill-seekers.
   - D. Conditions on Mount Everest make it difficult to survive.

7. According to the passage, what makes thrill-seekers different from other people?
   A. They have no concern for their own safety.
   B. They experience fear differently than others.
   C. They have an obsession that clouds their judgment.
   D. They accumulate greater amounts of dopamine in the brain.
8. Choose the best summary of the passage.
   A. Thrill-seekers are people who crave excitement and intense experiences. Scientists believe that high levels of dopamine in the brain might explain why thrill-seekers are willing to take the risks they do. Without thrill-seekers, the world might be a very different place than it is now.
   B. Psychologists describe "thrill-seeking" as an urge to do dangerous things. Many thrill-seekers have tried to climb Mount Everest, but most have died trying to reach the summit. Scientists believe that low levels of dopamine in the brain might cause thrill-seeking behavior.
   C. Thrill-seekers engage in risky behavior to achieve a "high" that most people never experience. This is why they continue to climb Mount Everest, even though no one has ever survived the attempt. Many thrill-seekers take dopamine to suppress their fears when attempting dangerous feats.
   D. Psychologists believe that thrill-seekers are motivated by danger, but scientists have discovered that they are motivated by the "high" they experience from taking dopamine. Thrill-seekers have explored outer space, built civilizations, and developed advanced technologies.

ANSWERS TO REVIEW QUESTIONS

1. A—main idea
2. D—inferences
3. B—meaning of words in context
4. B—author's purpose
5. C—author's tone
6. C—fact and opinion
7. D—supporting detail
8. A—summary

Bibliography

Johnson B: *The reading edge*, ed 4, New York, NY, 2001, Houghton Mifflin.

VOCABULARY

Members of the health professions use specific terminology to ensure accurate, concise, and consistent communication among all persons involved in the provision of health care. Although the following list is made up of general vocabulary words, many of these words are also used in a healthcare context. Careful study and review of these words will help you understand more of what you read and improve your ability to communicate in a professional manner.

Abrasive *adjective*: Irritating; rude or unfriendly.
> *Example:* Jim has an *abrasive* tone, but he is quite friendly once you get to know him.

Abstain *verb*: To voluntarily refrain from something.
> *Example:* The dentist told me to *abstain* from solid food after having my tooth pulled.

Accountable *adjective*: Answerable; responsible for one's actions.
> *Example:* If you throw a party at my house, you will be *accountable* for any damages to the property.

Acute *adjective*: Severe or intense; sharp.
> *Example:* After surviving the car crash, the driver was in *acute* need of medical attention.

Adhere *verb*: To hold fast or stick together.
> *Example:* If you want to play the game, you have to *adhere* to the rules.

Adjacent *adjective*: Close to; nearby.
> *Example:* The uncontrolled blaze posed a danger to the *adjacent* buildings.

Adverse *adjective*: Undesired, possibly harmful.
> *Example:* The event was cancelled due to *adverse* weather conditions.

Alleviate *verb*: To make less severe; to relieve.
> *Example:* Alex ate an apple to *alleviate* his hunger.

Ambiguous *adjective*: Of uncertain meaning; having more than one possible interpretation.
> *Example:* The psychic's predictions were *ambiguous*; they could mean almost anything.

Ambulate *verb*: To walk.
> *Example:* Fred was able to *ambulate* fairly well, but he had trouble going up and down the stairs.

Analogous *adjective*: Comparable, similar.
> *Example:* The abacus is an ancient counting device that is *analogous* to our modern calculators.

Anemic *adjective*: Weak; lifeless.
> *Example:* The comedian was discouraged by the *anemic* response to his jokes.

Anomaly *noun*: Something abnormal or unusual.
> *Example:* Beverly's failing grade was an *anomaly*; she has always been an excellent student.

Apathy *noun*: Lack of concern or interest.
> *Example:* Ever since Tim lost his job, his *apathy* toward finding a new one has increased.

Articulate *verb*: To speak clearly; to put into words.
> *Example:* Rob was too angry to *articulate* his thoughts without shouting.

Assert *verb*: To state something strongly.
> *Example:* You should not *assert* an opinion without backing it up with facts.

Atrophy *verb*: To gradually weaken due to lack of use or neglect.
> *Example:* The longer they were apart, the more their feelings for each other began to *atrophy*.

Audible *adjective*: Able to be heard.
> *Example:* I could see her lips move, but her voice was not *audible*.

Benevolent *adjective*: Kind-hearted; generous.
> *Example:* The *benevolent* king was slow to anger and quick to forgive.

Benign *adjective*: Harmless; gentle.
> *Example:* The wise old philosopher had a kind face and a *benign* smile.

Bilateral *adjective*: Present on two sides.
> *Example:* The *bilateral* peace treaty states that both countries must withdraw their troops from the region.

Bore *verb*: To make a hole by digging or drilling.
> *Example:* The miners spent several weeks trying to *bore* through the face of the mountain.

Cavity *noun*: An opening or an empty area.
> *Example:* The bluebird nested in a small *cavity* in the old willow tree.

Cerebral *adjective*: Intelligent; relating to the brain or the mind.
> *Example:* Instead of playing sports, Deborah enjoyed more *cerebral* games like chess.

Chronic *adjective*: Lasting or recurring over a long period of time.
> *Example:* Fred covers his desk with post-it notes to remedy his *chronic* forgetfulness.

Coherent *adjective*: Easy to understand; reasonable.
> *Example:* The author's *coherent* writing style made complicated subjects easy to understand.

Compensate *verb*: To make up for a fault or deficiency; to pay for something.

Example: James' work ethic and positive attitude helped *compensate* for his lack of experience.

Comprehend *verb*: To understand.

Example: I cannot *comprehend* how you are always late for class when you live only two blocks from school.

Concave *adjective*: Rounded inward.

Example: The *concave* roof was designed to collect rainwater for thirsty crops.

Concise *adjective*: Brief, to the point.

Example: We didn't understand why Sam wanted to quit the team, so he gave us a clear and *concise* explanation.

Congenital *adjective*: Making up an essential part of a person's character; natural.

Example: Emily was very generous and well-known for her *congenital* kindness.

Conspicuous *adjective*: Obvious; very noticeable.

Example: Henry looked very *conspicuous* when he arrived at the picnic wearing a tuxedo.

Constricted *adjective*: Limited or reduced.

Example: Dawn moved away from home because she felt *constricted* by her parents' rules.

Contingent *adjective*: Dependent.

Example: Maria's willingness to sell me her car was *contingent* on my ability to pay for it.

Copious *adjective*: Great in amount or number; heavy.

Example: The tropical storm produced *copious* amounts of rain.

Cursory *adjective*: Quick, perfunctory, not thorough.

Example: Lisa gave the menu a *cursory* glance before ordering her usual breakfast.

Debacle *noun*: Total failure; disaster.

Example: The concert turned into a *debacle* when the singer forgot the words to his songs.

Deficit *noun*: A deficiency or lack of something.

Example: The new uniforms cost more than expected, so the team held a fundraiser to cover the *deficit*.

Depleted *adjective*: Reduced; weakened or worn out.

Example: German fighting forces were *depleted* after their defeat at Stalingrad.

Deteriorate *verb*: To decline or worsen.

Example: What started out as a friendly debate would soon *deteriorate* into an angry shouting match.

Diffuse *adjective*: Spread over a large area; generalized.

Example: The setting sun produced a *diffuse* red glow along the horizon.

Dilute *verb*: To weaken or lessen.

Example: Printing too much money will *dilute* the value of our currency.

Discrete *adjective*: Distinct, separate.

Example: Jack and Kevin are identical twins, but they have *discrete* personalities.

HESI Hint

Discrete and *discreet* are commonly confused words. Discreet is used to describe someone who is polite and careful not to offend others.

Distend *verb*: To enlarge or expand.

Example: The new spending bill will only *distend* the city's already bloated budget.

Docile *adjective*: Easily controlled; agreeable.

Example: Some students objected to the new dress code, but most were *docile* and quick to comply.

Dormant *adjective*: Inactive; sleeping.

Example: People who live near the *dormant* volcano are afraid it might become active again.

Elicit *verb*: To cause a reaction; to draw out a response or emotion from someone.

Example: The photographer made funny faces to *elicit* a smile from the grumpy child.

Emit *verb*: To make a sound; to release something into the air.

Example: My dog began to *emit* whining noises as the storm grew louder.

Enhance *verb*: To increase or improve.

Example: Randall reads lots of books to *enhance* his knowledge of history.

Equilibrium *noun*: A state of balance.

Example: To have a successful career, one must find a happy *equilibrium* between work and family life.

Evasive *adjective*: Seeking to avoid or escape a situation.

Example: Marilyn was *evasive* about why she was late for work.

Evolve *verb*: To develop gradually.

Example: New communication technology has caused businesses to *evolve* over the past several years.

Exacerbate *verb*: To make worse or more severe.
 Example: An extended drought will damage farmlands and *exacerbate* our food shortages.

Fatal *adjective*: Resulting in death; causing failure or ruin.
 Example: The star player's injury dealt a *fatal* blow to their chances of winning the game.

Fatigue *noun*: Extreme tiredness; exhaustion.
 Example: After hiking up the steep hill, my legs gave out due to *fatigue*.

Febrile *adjective*: Extremely excited or active.
 Example: Thousands of *febrile* fans rushed onto the field after the team's exciting victory.

Flaccid *adjective*: Weak or soft.
 Example: Our powerful offense easily overcame the other team's *flaccid* defense.

Formidable *adjective*: Causing fear or awe.
 Example: Learning a new language is a *formidable* but rewarding challenge.

Fortify *verb*: To strengthen or build up.
 Example: The city added more cameras outside the courthouse to *fortify* the security system.

Futile *adjective*: Ineffective; useless.
 Example: Pete made a *futile* attempt to assemble his new furniture before reading the instructions.

Gratuitous *adjective*: Beyond what is necessary or appropriate.
 Example: Carl needed a second job to support his *gratuitous* spending habits.

Impair *verb*: To make weaker; to harm or damage.
 Example: A lack of sleep can *impair* your ability to think clearly.

Impede *verb*: To slow something down; to interfere with something.
 Example: Buying a new car right now will *impede* your ability to pay off your credit cards.

Impending *adjective*: Occurring in the near future, about to happen.
 Example: People rushed to buy food when they heard about the *impending* snowstorm.

Implied *verb*: Suggested without explicitly stating.
 Example: He *implied* that he was angry with me by refusing to answer my phone calls.

Inferred *verb*: Reached an opinion through reasoning.
 Example: I *inferred* that he was angry with me when he refused to answer my phone calls.

HESI Hint

The terms *imply* and *infer* are often confused and used interchangeably, but they do not have the same meaning. Remember: The sender of a message *implies*, and the receiver of the message *infers*.

Infirm *adjective*: Lacking strength; sick.
 Example: The aging actor was so *infirm* that he could not attend his own movie premiere.

Inflame *verb*: To cause intense excitement or anger.
 Example: If you can't control your emotions, you will only *inflame* the situation.

Infuse *verb*: To put into; to fill with something.
 Example: The teacher's main goal was to *infuse* the students with a passion for learning.

Ingest *verb*: To consume or absorb information.
 Example: This vocabulary lesson includes too many words to *ingest* in only a day.

Innate *adjective*: Natural; existing from birth.
 Example: Dogs have an *innate* ability to sense danger.

Insidious *adjective*: Gradually and secretly causing harm.
 Example: Social media is a powerful tool, but it can have *insidious* effects on a person's mental health.

Instill *verb*: To add something gradually.
 Example: The best way for a manager to *instill* loyalty among employees is to lead by example.

Insulate *verb*: To protect from harm by separating or isolating something.
 Example: The clever accountant created a phony corporation to *insulate* his boss from potential lawsuits.

Intact *adjective*: Complete; without any damage or harm.
 Example: Despite the disappointing loss, the team's confidence remained *intact*.

Intermittent *adjective*: Stopping and starting over time.

Example: The weather forecast called for *intermittent* thunderstorms.

Invasive *adjective*: Interfering, nosy.

Example: Robert's attempt to listen in on our private conversation was *invasive* and unwelcome.

Kinetic *adjective*: Energetic; lively.

Example: The band gave a *kinetic* performance that left the audience cheering for more.

Latent *adjective*: Present but not active or visible; undeveloped.

Example: Molly's trip to Mexico rekindled her *latent* desire to learn Spanish.

Lethargic *adjective*: Sluggish; lacking energy.

Example: After the 12-hour flight, I was too *lethargic* to go to the beach.

Malleable *adjective*: Easily changed; flexible.

Example: Roger had already decided whom he would vote for, but my opinion was still *malleable*.

Melancholy *noun*: A state of sadness or depression.

Example: Many people experience *melancholy* during the dark winter months.

Meticulous *adjective*: Thorough; careful to notice small details.

Example: Marty has a messy house, but he takes *meticulous* care of his lawn.

Migrate *verb*: To move or transfer.

Example: The decline of industry in the north caused many workers to *migrate* to the southern states.

Mitigate *verb*: To relieve or make something less severe or painful.

Example: Beth drank plenty of water to *mitigate* the effects of the intense heat.

Myopic *adjective*: Short-sighted.

Example: The *myopic* party planner failed to order enough food for unexpected guests.

Myriad *adjective*: Great in number; countless.

Example: The charming village featured *myriad* shops and restaurants for tourists to enjoy.

Nebulous *adjective*: Unclear; uncertain.

Example: Ray hasn't been accused of any crimes, and the reasons for his arrest are *nebulous*.

Negligible *adjective*: Small, slight, or unimportant.

Example: The wage increase is expected to have a *negligible* impact on company profits.

Obscure *adjective*: Difficult to see or understand; mysterious.

Example: The methods used to build the Great Pyramid of Giza remain *obscure*.

Obtuse *adjective*: Slow to understand; lacking sharpness.

Example: I'm sorry for being *obtuse*, but I need you to repeat the instructions once again.

Occluded *adjective*: Closed or obstructed.

Example: The entrance to the cave was partly *occluded* by rocks after the landslide.

Opaque *adjective*: Difficult to see through or understand.

Example: I've read the poem several times, but its meaning remains *opaque* to me.

Overt *adjective*: Obvious or easily observed.

Example: The workers' strike was an *overt* act of rebellion against unsafe working conditions.

Pacify *verb*: To sooth or calm.

Example: The manager offered a full refund to *pacify* the unhappy customers.

Palpable *adjective*: Easily felt or perceived.

Example: The jury was ready to announce the verdict, and the tension in the room was *palpable*.

Perpetual *adjective*: Constant; lasting forever.

Example: Because of her *perpetual* fear of sharks, Amy will never go swimming in the ocean.

Plethora *noun*: A large amount.

Example: The ice cream shop offered a *plethora* of different flavors.

Potent *adjective*: Producing a strong effect.

Example: Regular exercise is a *potent* remedy for stress.

Precipitous *adjective*: Very steep; rapid.

Example: The actor's fast rise to fame was followed by an equally *precipitous* fall.

Predisposed *adjective*: Willing or inclined to do something.

Example: Animals with lots of fur are *predisposed* to survive in colder temperatures.

Prodigious *adjective*: Extremely large in amount or size.

Example: A *prodigious* amount of money was donated to build the new library.

Profound *adjective*: Deep; possessing great knowledge or understanding.

Example: The speaker shared many *profound* insights about the impact of AI on healthcare technology.

Profusely *adverb*: In large amounts.
  Example: George began sweating *profusely* as he carried the heavy boxes up the stairs.
Proliferate *verb*: To spread or grow rapidly.
  Example: The CEO of the company resigned as rumors of a scandal began to *proliferate*.
Prolific *adjective*: Very productive or fruitful.
  Example: Germany is the most *prolific* exporter of automobiles in the world.
Rationale *noun*: An underlying reason.
  Example: Please explain your *rationale* for wanting to quit school and join the circus.
Recumbent *adjective*: Lying down; resting.
  Example: I wanted to get to school early, but my *recumbent* brother refused to get out of bed.
Recur *verb*: To occur again.
  Example: The doctor said my symptoms will *recur* if I stop taking the medicine.
Redundant *adjective*: More than what is needed; consisting of unnecessary repetition.
  Example: It would be *redundant* to fire an employee who has already decided to quit.
Residual *adjective*: Remaining, continuing.
  Example: The mold in our basement was caused by *residual* water from last year's flood.
Resuscitate *verb*: To revive or bring back to life.
  Example: Financial experts worked on a plan to *resuscitate* the lifeless economy.
Sanguine *adjective*: Hopeful; cheerful.
  Example: Despite some financial troubles, Paul remained *sanguine* about the future of his company.
Saturated *adjective*: Completely filled with something.
  Example: The witness's testimony was *saturated* with half-truths and outright lies.
Stagnate *verb*: To stop developing or progressing.

  Example: If you don't spend more time practicing the violin, your skills will *stagnate*.
Stoic *adjective*: Showing no emotions.
  Example: Thomas was a *stoic* child; his parents could never tell if he was happy or sad.
Supplement *verb*: To add something in order to make something else better.
  Example: Betty is looking for part-time work to *supplement* her income.
Suppress *verb*: To stop or subdue.
  Example: Steven tried to *suppress* his fear of public speaking by taking an acting class.
Tenuous *adjective*: Weak; uncertain.
  Example: As the last votes were being counted, the frontrunner held a *tenuous* lead over his surging opponent.
Toxic *adjective*: Causing harm, poisonous.
  Example: Tom's short temper had a *toxic* effect on all his relationships.
Ubiquitous *adjective*: Happening or appearing everywhere.
  Example: Since the mid-2000s, superhero movies have become *ubiquitous*.
Virulent *adjective*: Extremely harmful or severe.
  Example: The candidate launched a *virulent* attack on his opponent's character.
Visceral *adjective*: Based on strong emotions or instincts.
  Example: The singer's stunning performance earned a *visceral* reaction from the audience.
Vital *adjective*: Essential.
  Example: Protein is a *vital* part of a healthy diet.
Volatile *adjective*: Unstable; rapidly changing.
  Example: Ron is emotionally *volatile*; he might be laughing one minute and crying the next.

REVIEW QUESTIONS

1. Select the meaning of the underlined word in the sentence. The aging athlete wanted to resuscitate his career as a baseball player.
   A. Begin
   B. Revive
   C. Reconsider
   D. Finish

2. Select the meaning of the underlined word in the sentence. It will take some time to ingest all the information I just read.
   A. Absorb
   B. Repeat
   C. Summarize
   D. Explain

3. What word meaning "rapid or steep" best completes the sentence? Bad customer reviews caused a _____ decline in business for the restaurant.
   A. Precipitous
   B. Conspicuous
   C. Gratuitous
   D. Ubiquitous

4. What is the best definition of the word *occluded*?
   A. Expanded
   B. Unstable
   C. Weak
   D. Closed

5. Select the meaning of the underlined word in the sentence. An <u>acute</u> shortage of chickens has led to a limited supply of eggs.
   A. Mild
   B. Temporary
   C. Severe
   D. Permanent

6. Which word means the same as the underlined word in the sentence? To <u>lessen</u> the cost of fixing his roof, Daniel did most of the work himself.
   A. Stagnate
   B. Exacerbate
   C. Mitigate
   D. Compensate

7. Which is the correct definition of the word *malleable*?
   A. Inflexible
   B. Flexible
   C. Certain
   D. Uncertain

8. Select the meaning of the underlined word in the sentence. I took a <u>cursory</u> look at John's résumé before I hired him for the job.
   A. Curious
   B. Quick
   C. Necessary
   D. Careful

9. Select the meaning of the underlined word in the sentence. I invited Jim to come with us, but he was too <u>infirm</u> to go hiking up a mountain.
   A. Busy
   B. Old
   C. Sick
   D. Tired

10. Select the meaning of the underlined word in the sentence. Instead of becoming angry and frustrated, Lindsay took a <u>cerebral</u> approach to her problems.
    A. Positive
    B. Confident
    C. Original
    D. Intelligent

ANSWERS TO REVIEW QUESTIONS

1. B—Revive
2. A—Absorb
3. A—Precipitous
4. D—Closed
5. C—Severe
6. C—Mitigate

7. B—Flexible
8. B—Quick
9. C—Sick
10. D—Intelligent

GRAMMAR

In the United States, the ability to speak and write the English language using proper grammar is a sign of an educated individual. When people are sick and need information or care from individuals in the health professions, they expect healthcare workers to be professional, well-educated individuals. It is therefore imperative that everyone in the healthcare professions understands and uses proper grammar.

Grammar varies a great deal from language to language. English as a second language (ESL) students have an added burden to becoming successful. For example, nursing research literature indicates that ESL nursing students are at greater risk for attrition and failure of the licensing examination. However, this burden can be overcome by learning proper grammar.

CHAPTER OUTLINE

KEY TERMS

This chapter describes the parts of speech, important terms and their uses in grammar, commonly occurring grammatical errors, and suggestions for successful use of grammar.

HESI Hint

If English is your second language, listen only to English-speaking radio and television. If at all possible, speak only English at home and with friends.

Eight Parts of Speech

The eight parts of speech are nouns, pronouns, adjectives, verbs, adverbs, prepositions, conjunctions, and interjections.

Noun

A **noun** is a word or group of words that names a person, place, thing, or idea.

Common Noun A common noun is the general, not the particular, name of a person, place, or thing (e.g., *teacher, school, pencil*).

Proper Noun A proper noun is the official name of a person, place, or thing (e.g., *Fred, Paris, Washington University*). Proper nouns are capitalized.

Abstract Noun An abstract noun is the name of a quality or a general idea (e.g., *persistence, democracy*).

Collective Noun A collective noun is a noun that represents a group of persons, animals, or things (e.g., *family, flock, furniture*).

Pronoun

A **pronoun** is a word that takes the place of a noun, another pronoun, or a group of words acting as a noun. The word or group of words to which a pronoun refers is called the *antecedent*.

The *students* wanted *their* test papers graded and returned to *them* in a timely manner.

The word *students* is the antecedent of the pronouns *their* and *them*.

Personal Pronoun A personal pronoun refers to a specific person, place, thing, or idea by indicating the person speaking (first person), the person or people spoken to (second person), or any other person, place, thing, or idea being talked about (third person).

Personal pronouns also express number in that they are either singular or plural.

We (first person plural) were going to ask *you* (second person singular) to give *them* (third person plural) a ride to the office.

Possessive Pronoun A possessive pronoun is a form of personal pronoun that shows possession or ownership.

- That is *my* book.
- That book is *mine*.
- That is *his* book.
- That book is *his*.

A possessive pronoun does not contain an apostrophe.

HESI Hint

Do **not** use pronouns ending in *self* where they are inappropriate or unnecessary. Use endings with *self* or *selves* only when there is a noun or personal pronoun in the sentence to relate back to.

- I myself did the entire project.
- Sara did the entire project herself.

Notice that there are no such words as *hisself, theirself,* or *theirselves*.

Adjective

An **adjective** is a word, phrase, or clause that modifies a noun (the *biology* book) or pronoun (He is *nice*.). It answers the question *what kind* (a *hard* test), *which one* (an *English* test), *how many* (*three* tests), or *how much* (*many* tests). Verbs, pronouns, and nouns can act as adjectives. A type of verb form that functions as an adjective is a **participle**, which usually ends in *-ing* or *-ed*. Adjectives usually precede the noun or noun phrase that they modify (e.g., *the absent-minded professor*).

Examples

Verbs: The *scowling* professor, the *worried* student, the *broken* pencil

Pronouns: *My* book, *your* class, *that* book, *this* class

Nouns: The *professor's* class, the *biology* class

HESI Hint

Do **not** use the word *more* with certain adjectives, for example, those ending in *er*. It is improper grammar to say or to write *more better* or *more harder*. Likewise, do **not** use the word *most* with adjectives that end in *-est* or *-st*. It is improper grammar to say *most easiest* or *most worst*.

Verb

A **verb** is a word or phrase that is used to express an action or a state of being. A verb is the critical element of a sentence. Verbs express time through a property called *tense*. The three primary tenses are:

- Present—Mary *works*
- Past—Mary *worked*
- Future—Mary *will work*

Some verbs are known as "linking verbs" because they link, or join, the subject of the sentence to a noun, pronoun, or predicate adjective. A linking verb does not show action.

- The most commonly used linking verbs are forms of the verb *to be: am, is, are, was, were, being, been* (e.g., That man *is* my professor.).
- Linking verbs are sometimes verbs that relate to the five senses: *look, sound, smell, feel,* and *taste* (e.g., That exam *looks* difficult.).
- Sometimes linking verbs reflect a state of being: *appear, seem, become, grow, turn, prove,* and *remain* (e.g., The professor *seems* tired.).

HESI Hint

The *subjunctive mood* is used when referring to hypothetical situations or when expressing a wish or demand. Note the following verb changes that occur with the subjunctive mood.
- It is important that Vanessa send [**not** *sends*] her resumé immediately.
- I wish I were [**not** *was*] that smart.
- If I were [**not** *was*] you, I'd leave now.

Adverb

An **adverb** is a word, phrase, or clause that modifies a verb, an adjective, or another adverb.

Examples

Verb: He ate his lunch *quickly.*
Adjective: The dancer wears *very* colorful costumes.
Another Adverb: The student scored *quite* badly on the test.

Preposition

A **preposition** is a word that shows the relationship of a noun or pronoun to some other word in the sentence. A compound preposition is a preposition that is made up of more than one word. A prepositional phrase is a group of words that begins with a preposition and ends with a noun or a pronoun, which is called the *object* of the preposition. Box 4.1 lists commonly used prepositions.

Box 4.1 Commonly Used Prepositions

aboard	among
about	around
above	as
across	at
after	barring
against	before
along	behind
amid	below
	beneath
	beside
	between
	beyond
	but (except)
	by
	concerning
	considering
	despite
	down
	during
	except
	following
	for
	from
	in
	including
	inside
	into
	like
	minus
	near
	of
	off
	on
	onto
	opposite
	out
	outside
	over
	past
	pending
	plus
	prior to
	throughout
	to
	toward
	under
	underneath
	unlike
	until
	up
	upon
	with
	within
	without

Examples: Prepositional Phrases

Sam left the classroom *at noon.*
The students learned the basics *of grammar.*

Conjunction

A **conjunction** is a word that joins words, phrases, or clauses. *Coordinating* conjunctions connect words, phrases, or clauses of equal importance. Words that serve as coordinating conjunctions are *and, but, or, so, nor, for,* and *yet* (e.g., Helen wanted to leave, *but* her friend wanted to stay.).

Correlative conjunctions work in pairs to join words or phrases (e.g., *Neither* the teacher *nor* her assistant could read the student's handwriting.).

HESI Hint

Correlative conjunctions always stay in the same pairs. Two common pairs are *neither* and *nor* and *either* and *or.* These pairs should not be mixed; it is incorrect to use *neither* with *or* and *either* with *nor.* An easy way to remember this is to think that the two words that start with the letter "n" always go together.

Sometimes, *subordinating* conjunctions (Box 4.2) join two clauses or thoughts.

In this example, the subordinating conjunction while is used to connect the two elements of the sentence:
Example: While the family was away on vacation, their house flooded.
While the family was away on vacation is dependent on the rest of the sentence to complete its meaning.

Interjection

An **interjection** is a word or phrase that expresses emotion or exclamation. It does not have any grammatical connection to the other words in the sentence (e.g., *Yikes,* that test was hard. *Whew,* that test was easy.).

Nine Important Terms to Understand

There are nine important terms to understand: Clause, direct object, indirect object, phrase, predicate, predicate adjective, predicate nominative, sentence, and subject.

Box 4.2 Commonly Used Subordinating Conjunctions

after
because
before
until
since
when

Clause

A **clause** is a group of words that has a subject and a predicate. An **independent (main) clause** expresses a complete thought and can stand alone as a sentence.
Example: The professor distributed the examinations as soon as the students were seated.
The professor distributed the examinations expresses a complete thought and can stand alone as a sentence.

A **dependent (subordinate) clause** begins with a subordinating conjunction and does not express a complete thought and therefore cannot stand alone as a sentence. *As soon as the students were seated* does not express a complete thought. It needs the independent clause to complete the meaning and form the sentence.

HESI Hint

Independent clauses are used to write simple and compound sentences. Dependent clauses are added to an independent clause to form complex or compound-complex sentences. When a sentence begins with a dependent clause, use a comma to set it apart from the independent clause. However, when the dependent clause is at the end of a sentence, it should not be preceded by a comma.
The students were late for class, because the bus was delayed at a train crossing. [Incorrect]
The students were late for class because the bus was delayed at a train crossing. [Correct]

Direct Object

A **direct object** is the person or thing that is directly affected by the action of the verb. A direct object answers the question *what* or *whom* after a transitive verb.

Example: The students watched the professor distribute the examinations.

The professor answers *whom* the students watched.

HESI Hint

> A *transitive* verb is a verb that acts on a direct object. In this sentence, the transitive verb *needs* acts on the direct object *gas*:
> My car needs gas.
> An *intransitive* verb does not act on a direct object. This sentence contains the intransitive verb *died*:
> My car died.

Indirect Object

An **indirect object** is the person or thing that is indirectly affected by the action of the verb. A sentence can have an indirect object only if it has a direct object. An indirect object answers the question *to whom, for whom, to what,* or *for what* after an action verb.

Indirect objects come between the verb and direct object.

Example: The professor gave his class the test results.

His class is the indirect object. It comes between the verb (gave) and the direct object (test results), and it answers the question to whom.

Phrase

A **phrase** is a group of two or more words that acts as a single part of speech in a sentence. A phrase can be used as a noun, an adjective, or an adverb. A phrase lacks a subject and predicate.

Predicate

A **predicate** is the part of the sentence that tells what the subject does or what is done to the subject. It includes the verb and all the words that modify the verb.

Predicate Adjective

A **predicate adjective** follows a linking verb and helps to explain the subject.

My professors are *wonderful.*

Predicate Nominative

A **predicate nominative** is a noun or pronoun that follows a linking verb and helps to explain or rename the subject.

Professors are *teachers.*

Sentence

A **sentence** is a group of words that expresses a complete thought. Every sentence has a subject and a predicate. There are four types of sentences.

Declarative A declarative sentence makes a statement.

Example: I went to the store.

Interrogative An interrogative sentence asks a question.

Example: Did you go to the store?

Imperative An imperative sentence makes a command or request.

Example: Go to the store.

Exclamatory An exclamatory sentence makes an exclamation.

Example: You went to the store!

HESI Hint

> Many imperative sentences do not seem to have subjects. An imperative sentence often has an implied subject. For example, when we say *Stop that now*, the subject of the sentence, *you*, is implied *(You stop that now).*

Subject

A **subject** is a word, phrase, or clause that names whom or what the sentence is about.

Ten Common Grammatical Mistakes

Subject-Verb Agreement

A subject must agree with its verb in number. A singular subject requires a singular verb. Likewise, a plural subject requires a plural verb.

Incorrect: The students (plural noun) *was* (singular verb) in a hurry to finish their assignment.

Correct: The students (plural noun) *were* (plural verb) in a hurry to finish their assignment.

There are times when the subject-verb agreement can be tricky to determine.

When the Subject and Verb Are Separated

Find the subject and verb and make sure they agree.

Incorrect: The *question* that appears on all of the tests *are* inappropriate.

Correct: The *question* that appears on all of the tests *is* inappropriate.

Ignore any intervening phrases or clauses. Ignore words such as *including, along with, as well as, together with, besides, except,* and *plus.*

Example: The *dean,* along with his classes, *is* going on a tour of the facility.
Example: The *deans,* along with their classes, *are* going on a tour of the facility.

When the Subject Is a Collective Noun

A collective noun is singular in form but plural in meaning. It is a noun that represents a group of persons, animals, or things (e.g., *family, audience, committee, board, faculty, herd, flock*).

If the group is acting as a single entity, use a singular verb.

Example: The *faculty agrees* to administer the test.

If the group is acting separately, use a plural verb.

Example: The *faculty are* not in agreement about which test to administer.

When the Subject Is a Compound Subject

Usually, when the subject consists of two or more words that are connected by the word *and,* the subject is plural and calls for a plural verb.

Example: The *faculty* and the *students are* in the auditorium.

When the subject consists of two or more singular words that are connected by the words *or, either/or, neither/nor,* or *not only/but also,* the subject is singular and calls for a singular verb.

Example: Neither the *student* nor the *dean was* on time for class.

When the subject consists of singular and plural words that are connected by the words *or, either/or, neither/nor,* or *not only/but also,* choose a verb that agrees with the subject that is closest to the verb.

Example: Either the *students* or the *teaching assistant is* responsible.

Comma in a Compound Sentence

A **compound sentence** is a sentence that has two or more independent clauses. Each independent clause has a subject and a predicate and can stand alone as a sentence. When two independent clauses are joined by a coordinating conjunction such as *and, but, or,* or *nor,* place a comma before the conjunction.

Example: The professor thought the test was too easy, *but* the students thought it was too hard.

Run-On Sentence

A **run-on sentence** occurs when two or more complete sentences are written as though they were one sentence.

Example: The professor thought the test was too easy the students thought it was too hard.

A comma splice is one type of run-on sentence. It occurs when two independent clauses are joined by only a comma.

Example: The professor thought the test was too easy, the students thought it was too hard.

The problem can be solved by replacing the comma with a dash, a semicolon, or a colon; by adding a coordinating conjunction; or by making two separate sentences.

Pronoun Case

Is it correct to say, "It was *me*" or "It was *I*"; "It must be *they*" or "It must be *them*"?

The correct pronoun to use depends on the pronoun's case. *Case* refers to the form of a noun or pronoun that indicates its relation to the other words in a sentence. There are three cases: *nominative (subjective), objective,* and *possessive.* The case of a personal pronoun depends on the pronoun's function in the sentence. The pronoun can function as a subject, a complement (predicate nominative, direct object, or indirect object), an object of a preposition, or a replacement for a possessive noun.

Examples: Pronoun Use

- When the pronoun is the subject
  Example: I studied for the examination.
  I is the subject of the sentence. Therefore, the nominative form of the pronoun is used.
- When pronouns are the subject in a compound subject
  Is it correct to say, **"He and I** went to the conference" or **"Him and me** went to the conference"?
  Is it correct to say, **"John and me** worked through the night" or **"John and I** worked through the night"?

Is it correct to say, **"Her and Maria** liked the chocolate-covered toffee" or **"She and Maria** liked the chocolate-covered toffee"?

If we understand how the pronouns are used in each sentence, we know to use the nominative case. In the first example, *He and I* is correct; in the second example, *John and I* is correct; in the third example, *She and Maria* is correct.

HESI Hint

When choosing a pronoun that is part of a compound subject, sometimes it is helpful to say the sentence without the conjunction and the other subject. We would not say, **Him** *went to the conference* or **Me** *worked through the night* or **Her** *liked the chocolate-covered toffee*. However, we would say, **He** *went to the conference*, **I** *worked through the night*, and **She** *liked the chocolate-covered toffee*.

HESI Hint

It is considered polite to place the pronoun *I* last in a series: *Luke, Jo, and I strive to do a good job.*

- When the pronoun is the object of the preposition
  Example: Susan gave the results of the test to them.

  The pronoun *them* is the object of the preposition *to*. When the object of the preposition is a compound object, as in *"Susan gave the results of the test to Jo and me,"* the objective form of the pronoun is used.
- When the pronoun replaces a possessive noun
  Example: That desk is hers.

  The possessive pronoun *hers* is used to replace a possessive noun. For example, suppose there is a desk that belongs to Holly. We would say,
  That desk belongs to Holly. That is Holly's desk. That desk is Holly's. That desk is *hers*.

HESI Hint

Do not use an apostrophe with a possessive pronoun. There are no such words as *her's* or *their's*.

Pronouns That Indicate Possession

Personal pronouns have their own possessive forms, as shown in Table 4.1. Do not confuse these possessive pronouns with contractions that are

Table 4.1 Possessive Personal Pronouns

Pronoun	POSSESSIVE FORMS	
I	My	Mine
He	His	His
She	Her	Hers
We	Our	Ours
You	Your	Yours
They	Their	Theirs
It	Its	Its

similarly pronounced or spelled. Examples are shown in Table 4.2.

Incorrect Apostrophe Usage

Apostrophes are used to show possession or to show that letters have been omitted (i.e., a contraction). Apostrophes are **not** used to make words plural.

Examples of plurals: during the 1980s, from the Smiths, with the Inezes

Examples of possessives:

Singular: 1980's highest grossing film, Mr. Smith's home, Inez's car

Plural: the 1980s' highest grossing film, the Smiths' home, the Inezes' cars

Commas in a Series

Use commas to separate three or more items in a series or list. A famous dedication makes the problem apparent: "To my parents, Ayn Rand and God." Because of the comma placement, it appears as though Ayn Rand and God are the parents. Place a comma between each item in the list and before the conjunction to avoid confusion.

Example: The nursing student took classes in English, biology, and chemistry.

Table 4.2 Common Possessive Pronouns and Similar Contractions

Possessive Pronoun	Contraction
Its (belonging to *it*)	It's (it is, it has)
Their (belonging to *them*)	They're (they are)
Whose (belonging to *whom*)	Who's (who is, who has)
Your (belonging to *you*)	You're (you are)

Unclear or Vague Pronoun Reference

An unclear or vague pronoun reference makes a sentence confusing and difficult to understand.
Example: The teacher and the student knew that she was wrong.

Who was wrong: the teacher or the student? The meaning is unclear. Rewrite the sentence to avoid confusion.
Revised: The teacher and the student knew that the *student* was wrong.

Sentence Fragments

Sentence fragments are incomplete sentences.
Example: While the students were taking the test.
The students were taking the test is a complete sentence. However, use of the word *while* turns it into a dependent clause. In order to make the fragment a sentence, it is necessary to supply an independent clause.
Revised: While the students were taking the test, the professor walked around the classroom.

HESI Hint

Other words that commonly introduce dependent clauses are *among, because, although,* and *however.*

Misplaced Modifier

Misplaced modifiers are words or groups of words that are not located properly in relation to the words they modify.
Example: I fear my teaching assistant may have discarded the test I was grading in the trash can.
Was the test being graded in the trash can?
The modifier *in the trash can* has been misplaced. The sentence should be rewritten so that the modifier is next to the word, phrase, or clause that it modifies.
Revised: I fear the test I was grading may have been discarded in the trash can by my teaching assistant.

One type of misplaced modifier is a dangling participial phrase. A **participial phrase** acts as an adjective and is formed by a participle, its object, and the object's modifiers. A participial phrase modifies the noun or pronoun that either directly precedes or follows the phrase. When the participial phrase directly precedes or follows a noun or pronoun that it does not modify, the phrase is called a *dangling participial phrase.*
Example: Taking all the evidence into account, a verdict was rendered by the jury.

The participial phrase *Taking all the evidence into account* is intended to modify the noun *jury;* however, because the phrase is placed closest to *verdict,* it appears to be modifying *verdict* instead of *jury.* Therefore, the sentence as it is written implies that the verdict took the all the evidence into account, which is incorrect.
Revised: Taking all the evidence into account, the jury rendered its verdict.

Five Suggestions for Success

Eliminate Clichés

Clichés are expressions or ideas that have lost their originality or impact over time because of excessive use. Examples of clichés are *blind as a bat, dead as a doornail, flat as a pancake, raining cats and dogs, keep a stiff upper lip, let the cat out of the bag, sick as a dog, take the bull by the horns, under the weather, white as a sheet,* and *you can't judge a book by its cover.*

Clichés should be avoided whenever possible because they are old, tired, and overused. If tempted to use a cliché, endeavor to rephrase the idea.

Eliminate Euphemisms

A **euphemism** is a mild, indirect, or vague term that has been substituted for one that is considered harsh, blunt, or offensive. In many instances, euphemisms are used in a sympathetic manner to shield and protect. Some people refuse to refer to someone who has died as "dead." Instead, they may say that the person has *passed away* or *departed.* Euphemisms should be eliminated, and we should try to speak and write more accurately and honestly using our own words whenever appropriate.

It is also essential to use accurate and anatomically correct language when referring to the body, a body part, or a bodily function. To do otherwise is unprofessional and tactless.

Eliminate Sexist Language

Sexist language refers to spoken or written styles that unnecessarily identify gender. Such language can suggest a sexist attitude on the part of the speaker or writer. In order to avoid stereotypes, try to use gender-neutral titles that do not specify a particular gender. Remember that inclusive language seeks to incorporate everyone who may be associated with a profession or group of people (e.g., use *police officer* instead of *policeman*).

HESI Hint

Attempts to eliminate sexist language may create grammatical problems if the word *his or her* is replaced with the word *their*. For example, *The teacher helps their students.* However, this is grammatically incorrect because *their* is a plural pronoun that is being used in place of a singular noun. If the gender of the teacher is known, it is appropriate to use *his* or *her*. *The teacher helped her students.* If the gender is not known, it is better to reword the sentence to avoid incorrect grammar as well as sexist language.
- Teachers help their students.
- The students are helped by their teacher.

Eliminate Profanity and Insensitive Language

Insensitive and obscene language can be insulting and cruel. What we say does make a difference. The nursery rhyme we learned in our youth, "Sticks and stones may break my bones, but words will never hurt me," is simply not true. Ask anyone who has been on the receiving end of language that is patronizing or demeaning. Because language constantly changes, sometimes we can be offensive without even realizing that we have committed a blunder. In the age of an "anything goes" attitude for television, music lyrics, and the Internet, it is difficult to know exactly what constitutes offensive language.

We need to be sensitive to language that excludes or emphasizes a person or group of people with reference to race, sexual orientation, age, gender, religion, or disability. We would all do well to remember another adage from childhood: The Golden Rule. Its message is clear: Respect the dignity of every human being and treat others as you would like to be treated.

Eliminate Textspeak

Textspeak is language that is often used in text messages, emails, and other forms of electronic communication; it consists of abbreviations, slang, emoticons, and acronyms. With the pervasiveness of social media and text messaging, the use of textspeak may be second nature. However, it is important to be aware of when it is creeping into all electronic communication. Although textspeak is acceptable in informal communication, it is inappropriate to use textspeak in formal communication, such as in academic and professional settings. Just as use of proper grammar is taken as a sign of intelligence, use of textspeak can be taken as a sign of laziness.

Fifteen Troublesome Word Pairs

Affect Versus Effect

Affect is normally used as a verb that means "to influence or to change" (The medication *affected* [changed] my daily routine.). As a noun, *affect* is an emotional response or disposition (Children with autism often have a flat *affect* [emotional response]).

Effect may be used as a noun or a verb. As a noun, it means "result or outcome" (The medication had a strange *effect* [result] on me). As a verb, it means "to bring about or accomplish" (As a result of the medication, I was able to *effect* [bring about] a number of changes in my life).

Among Versus Between

Use *among* to show a relationship involving more than two persons or things being considered as a group (The professor will distribute the textbooks *among* the students in his class).

Use *between* to show a relationship involving two persons or things (I sit *between* Holly and Jo in class), to compare one person or thing with an entire group (What is the difference between this book and other grammar books?), or to compare more than two things in a group if each is considered individually (I cannot decide *between* the chemistry class, the biology class, and the anatomy class).

Amount Versus Number

Amount is used when referring to things in bulk (The teacher had a huge *amount* of paperwork).

Number is used when referring to individual, countable units (The teacher had a *number* of papers to grade).

Good Versus Well

Good is an adjective. Use *good* before nouns (He did a *good* job) and after linking verbs (She smells *good*) to modify the subject. *Well* is usually an adverb. When modifying a verb, use the adverb *well* (She plays softball *well*). *Well* is used as an adjective only when describing someone's health (She is getting *well*).

HESI Hint

To say that you feel well implies that you are in good health. To say that you are good or that you feel good implies that you are in good spirits.

Bad Versus Badly

Apply the same rule for *bad* and *badly* that applies to good and well. Use *bad* as an adjective before nouns (He is a bad teacher) and after linking verbs (That smells bad) to modify the subject. Use *badly* as an adverb to modify an action verb (The student behaved *badly* in class).

HESI Hint

Do not use *badly* (or other adverbs) when using linking verbs that have to do with the senses. Say, "You felt *bad*." To say, "You felt *badly*" implies that something was wrong with your sense of touch. Say, "The mountain air smells wonderful." To say, "The mountain air smells wonderfully" implies that the air has a sense of smell that is used in a wonderful manner.

Bring Versus Take

Bring conveys action toward the speaker—to carry from a distant place to a near place (Please *bring* your textbooks to class).

Take conveys action away from the speaker—to carry from a near place to a distant place (Please *take* your textbooks home).

Can Versus May (Could Versus Might)

Can and *could* imply ability or power (I *can* get an A in that class). *May* and *might* imply permission (You *may* leave early) or possibility (I *might* leave early).

Farther Versus Further

Farther refers to a measurable distance (The walk to class is much *farther* than I expected). *Further*

refers to a figurative distance and means "to a greater degree" or "to a greater extent" (I will have to study *further* to make better grades). *Further* also means "moreover" (Further/Furthermore, let me tell you something) and "in addition to" (The student had nothing *further* to say).

Fewer Versus Less

Fewer refers to number—things that can be counted or numbered—and is used with plural nouns (The professor has *fewer* students in his morning class than in his afternoon class).

Less refers to degree or amount—things in bulk or in the abstract—and is used with singular nouns (*Fewer* students make *less* work for the teacher). *Less* is also used when referring to numeric or statistical terms (It is *less* than 2 miles to school. He scored *less* than 90 on the test. She spent *less* than $400 for this class. I am *less* than 5 feet tall.).

Hear Versus Here

Hear is a verb meaning "to recognize sound by means of the ear" (I *hear* the music playing). *Here* is most commonly used as an adverb meaning "at or in this place" (The test will be *here* tomorrow).

i.e. Versus e.g.

The abbreviation *i.e.* (that is) is often confused with *e.g.* (for example); *i.e.* specifies or explains (I love to study chemistry, *i.e.*, the science dealing with the composition and properties of matter), and *e.g.* gives an example (I love to study chemistry, *e.g.*, chemical equations, atomic structure, and molar relationships).

Learn Versus Teach

Learn means "to receive or acquire knowledge" (I am going to *learn* all that I can about math). *Teach* means "to give or impart knowledge" (I will *teach* you how to convert decimals to fractions).

Lie Versus Lay

Lie means "to recline or rest." The principal forms of the verb are *lie, lay, lain,* and *lying.* Because *lie* is an intransitive verb, forms of *lie* are never followed by a direct object.

Examples

- I will *lie* down and rest.
- I *lay* down yesterday to rest.
- I had *lain* down to rest.
- I was *lying* on the sofa.

Lay means "to put or place." The principal forms of the verb are *lay, laid, laid,* and *laying.* Because *lay* is a transitive verb, forms of *lay* require a direct object.

Examples

- I *lay* the book on the table.
- I *laid* the book on the table yesterday.
- I have *laid* the book on the table before.
- I am *laying* the book on the table now.

A summary of verb forms for *lie* and *lay* is shown in Table 4.3.

HESI Hint

To help determine whether the use of *lie* or *lay* is appropriate in a sentence, substitute the word in question with "place, placed, placing" (whichever is appropriate). If the substituted word makes sense, the equivalent form of *lay* is correct. If the sentence does not make sense with the substitution, the equivalent form of *lie* is correct.

Which Versus That

Which is used to introduce nonessential clauses, and *that* is used to introduce essential clauses. A nonessential clause adds information to the sentence but is not necessary to make the meaning of the sentence clear. Use commas to set off a nonessential clause. An essential clause adds information to the sentence that is needed to make the sentence clear. Do not use commas to set off an essential clause.

Example: The school, *which flooded last July*, is down the street.

In this case, the phrase *which flooded last July* is a nonessential clause that is simply providing more information about the school.

Example: The school *that flooded last July* is down the street; the other school is across town.

In this case, the phrase *that flooded last July* is an essential clause because the information distinguishes the two schools as the one that flooded and the one that did not.

Who Versus Whom

Who and *whom* serve as interrogative pronouns and relative pronouns. An interrogative pronoun is one that is used to form questions, and a relative pronoun is one that relates groups of words to nouns or other pronouns.

Examples

- *Who* is getting an A in this class? (Interrogative)
- Susan is the one *who* is getting an A in this class. (Relative)
- To *whom* shall I give the textbook? (Interrogative)
- Susan, *whom* the professor favors, is very bright. (Relative)
  Who and *whom* may be singular or plural.

Examples

- *Who* is getting an A in this class? (Singular)
- *Who* are the students getting As in this class? (Plural)
- *Whom* did you say is passing the class? (Singular)
- *Whom* did you say are passing the class? (Plural)
  Who is the nominative case. Use *who* for subjects and predicate nominatives (doers of the action).

HESI Hint

Use *who* or *whoever* if *he, she, they, I,* or *we* can be substituted in the *who* clause.

Who passed the chemistry test? *He/she/they/I* passed the chemistry test.

Whom is the objective case. Use *whom* for direct objects, indirect objects, and objects of the preposition (receivers of the action).

Table 4.3 Lay Versus Lie

Infinitive	Meaning	Present Tense	Past Tense	Present Participle	Past Participle
lie	to recline or rest	lie	lay	lain	lying
lay	to put or place	lay	laid	laid	laying

HESI Hint

Use *whom* or *whomever* if *him, her, them, me,* or *us* can be substituted as the object of the verb or as the object of the preposition in the *whom* clause.

To *whom* did the professor give the test? He gave the test to *him/her/them/me/us.*

Summary

Review this chapter and ask yourself whether your use of the English language reflects that of an educated individual. If so, congratulations! If not, study the content of this chapter, and your scores on the HESI Admission Assessment are likely to improve.

REVIEW QUESTIONS

1. Identify the type of grammatical error in the following sentence. After reading the final chapter, the book was returned to the library.
   A. Dangling participial phrase
   B. Comma splice
   C. Subject-verb agreement error
   D. Run-on sentence

2. Which word in the following sentence is an adverb? Although the line was long, Stephen patiently waited for his turn to ride the roller coaster.
   A. Although
   B. long
   C. patiently
   D. his

3. Which word in the following sentence is an indirect object? David wasn't hungry, so he gave me his sandwich.
   A. David
   B. me
   C. his
   D. sandwich

4. Which pronoun correctly completes the sentence? The CEO of the company, _____ we used to admire, was caught cheating on his taxes.
   A. who
   B. which
   C. that
   D. whom

5. Which of the following sentences is grammatically correct?
   A. She laid her head on the desk.
   B. My dog laid on the chair.
   C. The sick boy laid in bed.
   D. I laid down and went to sleep.

6. Select the best word for the blank in the following sentence. The organizer printed dozens of fliers and distributed them ___ all the volunteers.
   A. along
   B. among
   C. between
   D. beneath

7. Which word in the following sentence is a preposition? The musicians quickly tuned their instruments before the concert.
   A. The
   B. quickly
   C. their
   D. before

8. Which word in the following sentence should be replaced? A good doctor always listens to his patients.
   A. good
   B. always
   C. his
   D. patients

9. Select the best word for the blank in the following sentence. If you don't take the medication as directed, it will not have the desired _____ on your health.
   A. affect
   B. effect
   C. effectiveness
   D. affectiveness

10. What word is used incorrectly in this sentence? Its too soon to tell whether Janice's baby is a boy or a girl.
    A. Its
    B. too
    C. whether
    D. Janice's

ANSWERS TO REVIEW QUESTIONS

1. A—In this sentence, *after reading the final chapter* is a participial phrase that appears to modify *book*; however, the intended subject (the reader of the book) is missing from the sentence. This is an example of a dangling participial phrase.

2. C—*Patiently* is an adverb that modifies *waited*.

3. B—An indirect object is the person or thing indirectly affected by the action of the verb. Indirect objects come between the verb and the direct object. In this sentence, the indirect object *me* receives the direct object *sandwich*.

4. D—*Whom* is an objective case pronoun. In this sentence, *whom* is the object of the verb *admire*.

5. A—*Laid* is the past tense form of *lay*, which means "to lay something down." In this sentence, the verb *laid* acts on the direct object *head*.

6. B—In this sentence, *among* is correct because the fliers are being distributed to a group of people.

7. D—In this sentence, *before* is used as a preposition of time.

8. C—The use of the possessive pronoun *his* in this sentence is an example of sexist language. This problem can be avoided by making the subject (doctor) plural and employing a gender-neutral pronoun: *Good doctors always listen to their patients.*

9. B—The correct word for this sentence is *effect*, which is a noun that means "a result of something." *Affect* is most often used as a verb that means "to influence or to change."

10. A—*Its* is a possessive pronoun. The correct word for the beginning of this sentence is the contraction *It's*, meaning "it is."

BIOLOGY

5

Biology is the scientific study of life; therefore, comprehending its basic components is important for understanding injuries and diseases. This chapter reviews the structure of cells and molecules and describes some of the vital functions they perform. The concepts of cellular respiration, photosynthesis, cellular reproduction, protein synthesis, genetics, disease, and immunity are also presented.

CHAPTER OUTLINE

Biology Basics
Water
Homeostasis
The Cell
Metabolic Pathways

The Cell Cycle
Cellular Reproduction
Nucleic Acids: DNA and RNA
Protein Synthesis
Genetics

Infectious Diseases
The Immune System
Review Questions
Answers to Review Questions

KEY TERMS

Active Transport
Adaptive Immune System
Alleles
Amino Acids
Anticodon
Binary Fission
Cell
Chain of Infection
Chromosomes
Citric Acid Cycle (also called Krebs Cycle)
Codon
Concentration Gradient
Cytokinesis
Deoxyribonucleic Acid (DNA)

Electron Transport Chain
Genes
Germ Theory
Glycolysis
Golgi Apparatus
Heterozygous
Homeostasis
Homozygous
Innate Immune System
Interphase
Meiosis
Messenger RNA (mRNA)
Metabolic Pathway
Metaphase Plate
Mitosis

Negative Feedback
Organelles
Passive Transport
Phagocytosis
Phospholipids
Photosynthesis
Positive Feedback
Punnett Square
Ribonucleic Acid (RNA)
Rough Endoplasmic Reticulum (ER)
Smooth ER
Stop Codon
Transcription
Transfer RNA (tRNA)
Translation

Biology Basics

Taxonomy is a system for studying, naming, and classifying biological organisms. In the taxonomic ranking system, kingdom is the largest and most inclusive category, while species is the most restrictive category. The order is as follows:

- Kingdom
- Phylum

- Class
- Order
- Family
- Genus
- Species

Science is a process. For an experiment to be performed, the following steps (commonly called the Scientific Method) must be taken:

- The first step is observation. New observations are made and/or previous data are studied.
- The second step is hypothesis, which is a statement or explanation of certain events or happenings.
- The third step is the experiment, which is a repeatable procedure of gathering data to support or refute the hypothesis.
- The fourth step in the scientific process is the conclusion, which provides a full explanation of the data and its significance.

Water

All life, and therefore biology, occurs in a water-based (or aqueous) environment. The water molecule consists of two hydrogen atoms covalently bonded to one oxygen atom. The most significant aspect of water is the polarity of its bonds that allow for hydrogen bonding between molecules. This type of intermolecular bonding has several resulting benefits. The first of these is water's high specific heat.

Specific heat is the amount of heat necessary to raise the temperature of 1 gram of a substance by 1° Celsius. Water has a relatively high specific heat value due to the extent of hydrogen bonding between water molecules, which allows water to resist shifts in temperature. One powerful benefit is the ability of oceans or large bodies of water to stabilize climates.

Hydrogen bonding also results in strong cohesive and adhesive properties. Cohesion is the ability of a molecule to stay bonded or attracted to another molecule of the same substance. A good example is how water tends to run together on a newly waxed car. Adhesion is the ability of water to bond to or attract other molecules or substances. When water is sprayed on a wall, some of it sticks to the wall. That is adhesion.

When water freezes, it forms a crystal lattice. This causes the molecules to spread apart, resulting in the phenomenon of ice floating in water. Water is unique in this regard since most solids do not float on the liquid form of their substance because the molecules pack tighter in the solid form.

The polarity of water also allows it to act as a versatile solvent. Water can be used to dissolve a number of different substances (Fig. 5.1).

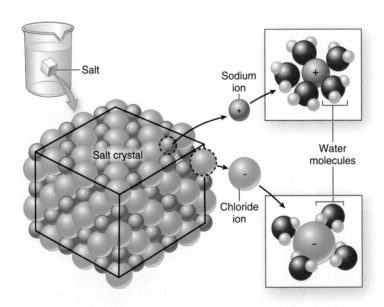

FIGURE 5.1　Water as a solvent. The polar nature of water *(blue)* favors ionization of substances in solution. Sodium (Na$^+$) ions *(pink)* and chloride (Cl−) ions *(green)* dissociate in the solution. (From Patton KT, Thibodeau GA: *Anatomy and physiology*, ed 9, St Louis, 2016, Mosby.)

Homeostasis

The human body is made up of *trillions* of cells that perform hundreds of functions. These cells work together to provide a relatively constant internal environment. An organism's ability to maintain a stable internal environment is called **homeostasis**. Homeostasis is responsible for maintaining many of the body's internal variables, such as blood pressure and body temperature. Under ideal conditions, these variables operate within a narrow range of values called a *set point*. When conditions in the environment cause values to move away from the set point (i.e., away from homeostasis), the body normally resists these changes through a mechanism called **negative feedback** (Fig. 5.2). A negative feedback loop is triggered when an abnormal variable produces a *stimulus*. The stimulus is measured by a *sensor*, which sends an error signal to a *control center*. The control center detects the error and sends this information to an *effector*, which produces a response that reduces the effect of the stimulus and restores the variable back to its set point. All systems under homeostatic regulation use negative feedback. In a few instances, the body responds to a stimulus by moving the variable further away from the set point, thereby increasing the effect of the stimulus. This is called **positive feedback**.

The Cell

The **cell** is the fundamental unit of biology. There are two types of cells: prokaryotic and eukaryotic. Cells consist of many components, most of which are referred to as **organelles**. Figure 5.3 illustrates a typical cell.

Prokaryotic cells lack a defined nucleus and do not contain membrane-bound organelles. Eukaryotic cells have a membrane-enclosed nucleus and a series of membrane-bound organelles that carry out the functions of the cell as directed by the genetic information contained in the nucleus. In other words, prokaryotic cells do not have membrane-bound organelles, whereas eukaryotic cells do. The eukaryotic cell is the more complex of the two cell types.

There are several different organelles functioning in a cell at a given time; only the major ones are considered here.

Nucleus

The first of the organelles is the nucleus, which contains the DNA of the cell in organized masses called **chromosomes.** Chromosomes contain all of the genetic information for the regeneration (repair and replication) of the cell, as well as all instructions for the function of the cell. Every organism has a characteristic number of chromosomes specific to the particular species.

Ribosomes

Ribosomes are organelles that read the RNA produced in the nucleus and translate the genetic instructions to produce proteins. Cells with a high rate of protein synthesis generally have a large number of ribosomes. Ribosomes can be found in two locations. Bound ribosomes are those found attached to the endoplasmic reticulum, and free ribosomes are those found in the cytoplasm. The two types are

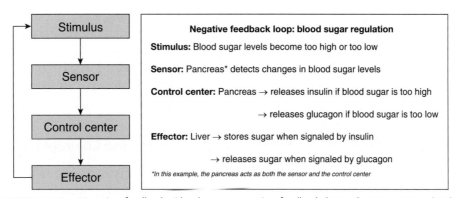

FIGURE 5.2 Negative feedback. Blood sugar negative feedback loop: the pancreas maintains glucose homeostasis by producing insulin and glucagon.

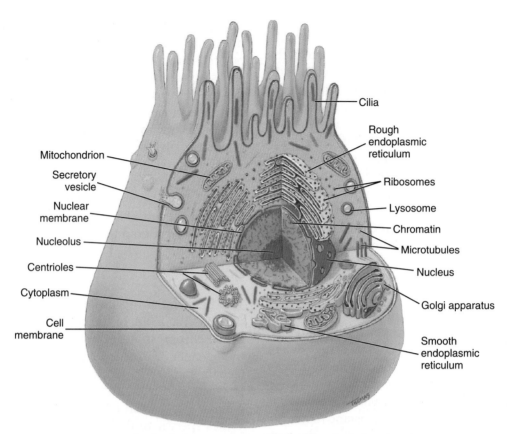

FIGURE 5.3 Generalized cell. (From Applegate: *The anatomy and physiology learning system,* ed 4, St Louis, 2011, Saunders.)

interchangeable and have identical structures, although they have slightly different roles.

Endoplasmic Reticulum

The endoplasmic reticulum (ER) is a membranous organelle that consists of two continuous parts. The first part extends from the nuclear membrane and is covered with ribosomes. This section of the ER is referred to as **rough ER**, and it is responsible for protein synthesis. The other section of the ER is continuous with the rough ER, but it lacks ribosomes. This part is referred to as **smooth ER**. Functions of the smooth ER include the synthesis of lipids, such as **phospholipids** and cholesterol that make up the cellular membrane, and the metabolism of carbohydrates. In liver cells, the smooth ER helps process the waste products of metabolism and aids in the detoxification of drugs and alcohol.

Golgi Apparatus

Inside the cell is a packaging, processing, and shipping organelle called the **Golgi apparatus.** The Golgi apparatus transports proteins from the ER throughout the cell.

Lysosomes

Intracellular digestion takes place in lysosomes. Packed with hydrolytic enzymes, lysosomes can hydrolyze proteins, fats, sugars, and nucleic acids. Lysosomes normally contain an acidic environment (around pH 4.5).

Vacuoles

Vacuoles are membrane-enclosed structures that have various functions, depending on cell type. Many cells, through a process called **phagocytosis,** uptake food through the cell membrane, creating a food vacuole. Plant cells have a central vacuole that is used for storage, waste disposal, protection, and hydrolysis.

Mitochondria and Chloroplasts

There are two distinct organelles that produce cell energy: the mitochondrion and the chloroplast. Mitochondria are found in most eukaryotic cells and are the site of cellular respiration. Chloroplasts are found in plants and are the site of photosynthesis.

Cellular Membrane

The cellular membrane is the most important component of the cell, contributing to protection, communication, and the passage of substances into and out of the cell. The cell membrane itself consists of a bilayer of phospholipids with proteins, cholesterol, and glycoproteins peppered throughout. The phospholipid heads, which are located on the external surfaces of the membrane, are hydrophilic (water loving). The fatty acid tails, which are located inside the membrane, are hydrophobic (water fearing). Membrane phospholipids are referred to as *amphipathic* because they have both hydrophilic and hydrophobic properties; this makes the cellular membrane selectively permeable.

Membrane Transport

Some substances pass through the cell membrane by **passive transport**, a method in which ions and molecules move along a **concentration gradient**. When there is a relatively high concentration of a substance on one side of the cell membrane, the substance tends to move to the other side of the membrane where there is less of that substance. Because passive transport occurs along the concentration gradient, no energy is used up. One type of passive transport is *simple diffusion*, which allows small nonpolar molecules to pass through the cell membrane without the help of membrane proteins. Simple diffusion of water across the cell membrane is called *osmosis*. *Facilitated diffusion* is a type of passive transport in which molecules move into and out of the cell with the help of transmembrane proteins (also called membrane channel proteins), which are proteins that pass through the cell membrane and act as transport highways for polar or charged molecules. Other molecules move in and out of the cell *against* a concentration gradient. This type of movement requires the expenditure of energy and is called **active transport**. Figure 5.4 illustrates the structure of the cellular membrane.

Metabolic Pathways

Metabolism is the sum of all chemical reactions that occur in an organism. In a cell, reactions take place in a series of steps called **metabolic pathways,** progressing from a standpoint of high energy to low energy. Metabolic processes may be either catabolic or anabolic. Catabolism is the process of breaking down complex molecules into simpler ones. Anabolism is the process of forming more complex molecules from smaller molecules. All of the reactions are catalyzed by the use of enzymes.

Cellular Respiration

There are two catabolic pathways that lead to cellular energy production. As a simple combustion reaction, cellular respiration produces far more energy than does its anaerobic counterpart, fermentation.

$$C_6H_{12}O_6 + 6O_2 \rightarrow 6CO_2 + 6H_2O$$

This balanced equation is the simplified chemistry behind respiration. The process itself actually occurs in a series of three complex steps that are simplified for our purposes.

The first stage in the metabolism of food to cellular energy is the conversion of glucose to pyruvate in a process called **glycolysis.** It takes place in the cytosol of the cell and produces two molecules of adenosine triphosphate (ATP), pyruvate, and nicotinamide adenine dinucleotide hydride (NADH) each. ATP provides the energy needed for metabolism and other processes in the cell. Pyruvate is a chemical compound that links glycolysis with other metabolic pathways. NADH acts as a reducing agent and is a vehicle of stored energy; this molecule is used as a precursor to produce greater amounts of ATP in the final steps of respiration.

In stage two, pyruvate is transported into a mitochondrion and is used in the first of a series of reactions called the **citric acid cycle** (also called the Krebs cycle). This cycle takes place in the matrix of the mitochondria, and it produces two ATP molecules, six carbon dioxide molecules, and six NADH molecules for each glucose molecule consumed.

The third stage is called the **electron transport chain**, which is located in the inner mitochondrial membrane. In this stage, electrons from NADH are transferred to electron carriers in the chain. The electrons are eventually transferred to oxygen in order to form water. The energy harvest here is remarkable. For every glucose molecule, 28 to 32 ATP molecules can be produced.

This conversion results in overall ATP production numbers of 32 to 36 ATP molecules for every glucose molecule consumed. For a summary of cellular respiration, see Figure 5.5.

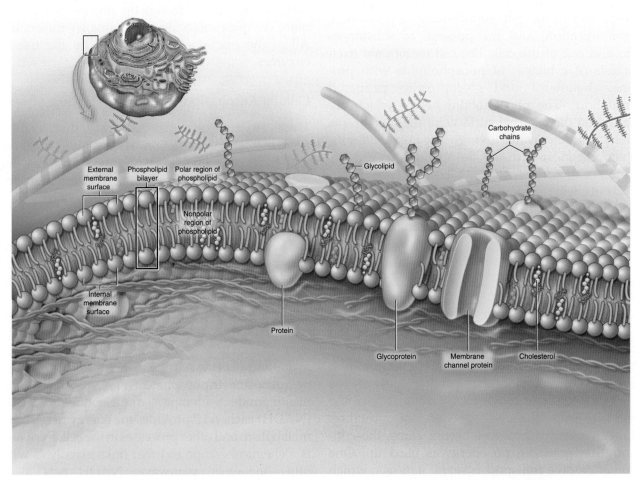

FIGURE 5.4   The plasma membrane is made of a bilayer of phospholipid molecules arranged with their nonpolar "tails" pointing toward each other. Cholesterol molecules help stabilize the flexible bilayer structure to prevent breakage. Protein molecules and protein-hybrid molecules may be found on the outer or inner surface of the bilayer—or extending all the way through the membrane. (From Patton KT, Thibodeau GA: *Anatomy and physiology*, ed 9, St Louis, 2016, Mosby.)

Photosynthesis

In the previous section, the harvesting of energy by the cell was discussed. But where did that energy originate? It began with a glucose molecule and resulted in a large production of energy in the form of ATP. A precursor to the glucose molecule is produced in a process called **photosynthesis**.

The chemical reaction representing this process is simply the reverse of cellular respiration.

$$6CO_2 + 6H_2O + \text{Light energy} \rightarrow C_6H_{12}O_6 + 6O_2$$

The only notable difference is the addition of light energy on the reactant side of the equation. Just as glucose is used to produce energy, so too must energy be used to produce glucose.

Photosynthesis is not as simple a process as it looks from the chemical equation. In fact, it consists of two different stages: the light reactions and the Calvin cycle. The light reactions are those that convert solar energy to chemical energy. The cell accomplishes the production of ATP by absorbing light and using that energy to split a water molecule and transfer the electron, thus creating nicotinamide adenine dinucleotide phosphate and producing ATP. These molecules are then used in the Calvin cycle to produce sugar.

The sugar produced is polymerized and stored as a polymer of glucose. These sugars are consumed by organisms or by the plant itself to produce energy by cellular respiration.

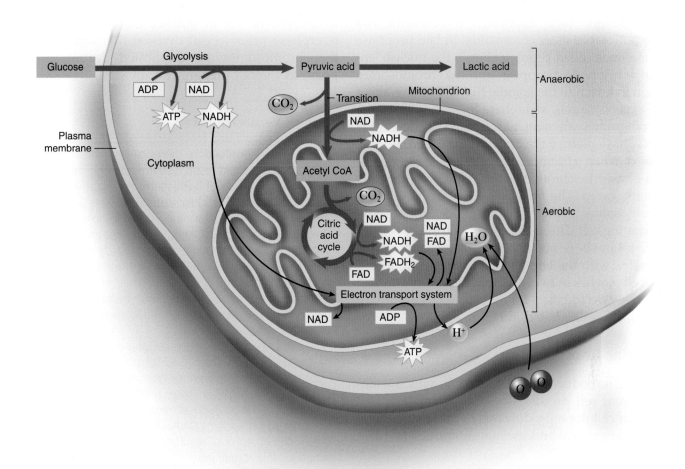

FIGURE 5.5 Summary of cellular respiration. This simplified outline of cellular respiration represents one of the most important catabolic pathways in the cell. Note that one phase *(glycolysis)* occurs in the cytosol but that the two remaining phases (*citric acid cycle* and *electron transport system*) occur within a mitochondrion. Note also the divergence of the *anaerobic* and *aerobic* pathways of cellular respiration. *ADP,* Adenosine diphosphate; *ATP,* adenosine triphosphate; *CoA,* coenzyme A; *FAD,* flavin adenine dinucleotide; *FADH₂,* form of flavin adenine dinucleotide; *NAD,* nicotinamide adenine dinucleotide; *NADH,* form of nicotinamide adenine dinucleotide. (From Patton KT, Thibodeau GA: *Anatomy and physiology,* ed 9, St Louis, 2016, Mosby.)

HESI Hint

When attempting to understand cell respiration and photosynthesis, keep in mind that these processes are cyclical. In other words, the raw materials for one process are the products of the other process. The raw materials for cellular respiration are glucose and oxygen, whereas the products of cell respiration are water, carbon dioxide, and ATP. Plants and other autotrophs will utilize the products of cell respiration (water, carbon dioxide) in the process of photosynthesis. The products of photosynthesis (oxygen, glucose) become the raw materials of cell respiration.

The Cell Cycle

The eukaryotic cell cycle is the process by which body cells (also called somatic cells) grow and divide. The two main phases of the cell cycle are **interphase** and **mitosis**. Interphase is the longest part of the cell cycle and is the phase during which the cell grows and replicates its DNA. Mitosis is the cell division phase. Mitosis occurs in four stages before pinching in two in a process called **cytokinesis**. The four stages are prophase, metaphase, anaphase, and telophase.

During prophase, the chromosomes are visibly separate, and each duplicated chromosome has two noticeable sister chromatids. In late prophase (sometimes called prometaphase), the nuclear envelope begins to disappear, and the chromosomes begin to attach to the spindle that is forming along the axis of the cell. Metaphase follows, with all the chromosomes aligning along what is called the **metaphase plate** or the center of the cell. Anaphase begins when chromosomes start to separate. In this phase, the chromatids are considered separate chromosomes. The final phase is telophase. Here, chromosomes gather on either side of the now separating cell. This is the end of mitosis.

Cytokinesis is not part of mitosis, although it overlaps with the late phases. During cytokinesis, the cell pinches in two, dividing the cytoplasm and forming two identical daughter cells. A summary of mitosis is illustrated in Figure 5.6.

Cellular Reproduction

Cellular reproduction is a process in which a single parent cell produces new daughter cells. All types of cellular reproduction fall into two general categories: sexual and asexual reproduction.

Asexual Reproduction

One type of asexual reproduction used by bacterial cells and other prokaryotes is called **binary fission.** In this process, the cell's single chromosome binds to the plasma membrane where it replicates. Then as the cell grows, it pinches in two, producing two identical cells (Fig. 5.7).

Sexual Reproduction

Sexual reproduction is different from asexual reproduction. In asexual reproduction, the offspring originates from a single cell, and all the cells produced are identical. In sexual reproduction, two cells contribute genetic material, resulting in significantly greater variation. These two cells find and fertilize each other randomly, making it virtually impossible for cells to be alike.

Meiosis is the process that produces sex cells (also called gametes). Meiosis consists of two distinct stages, meiosis I and meiosis II, resulting in four daughter cells (Fig. 5.8). Each of these daughter cells contains half as many chromosomes as the parent. As in mitosis, the cell undergoes interphase prior to cell division. Remember that the chromosomes are duplicated during interphase as the cell prepares for division.

HESI Hint

Meiosis Versus Mitosis

To illustrate the need for reduction division (meiosis I) in sexual cell production, calculate the chromosome numbers that would result if sperm and egg cells were produced by mitosis. If both sperm and eggs were the result of mitosis, their chromosome number would be 46, not 23. At fertilization, the chromosome number of the zygote would be 92, and the gametes produced by such an individual would also have 92 chromosomes. Of course, a zygote resulting from the fertilization of gametes containing 92 chromosomes would have a chromosome number of 184. The need to produce gametes by meiotic and not mitotic division soon becomes obvious.

Meiosis I consists of four phases: prophase I, metaphase I, anaphase I, and telophase I. The significant differences between meiosis and mitosis occur in prophase I. During this phase, nonsister chromatids of homologous chromosomes cross at numerous locations. Small sections of DNA are transferred between these chromosomes, resulting in increased genetic variation. The remaining three phases are the same as those in mitosis, with the exception that the chromosome pairs separate, not the chromosomes themselves.

After the first cytokinesis, meiosis II begins. All four stages of meiosis II are identical to those of mitosis. The resulting four cells have half as many chromosomes as the parent cell.

Nucleic Acids: DNA and RNA

Nucleic acids are chain-like macromolecules made up of building-block molecules called nucleotides. The two main types of nucleic acids are **deoxyribonucleic acid (DNA)** and **ribonucleic acid (RNA)**. DNA is a double helical structure with a backbone of alternating sugar and phosphate groups (Fig. 5.9). Each DNA molecule contains the unique genetic code that is necessary for replication. RNA carries genetic information from DNA to make the proteins that perform many of the cell's vital functions. The flow of genetic information from DNA to RNA to protein is known as the "central dogma" of molecular biology.

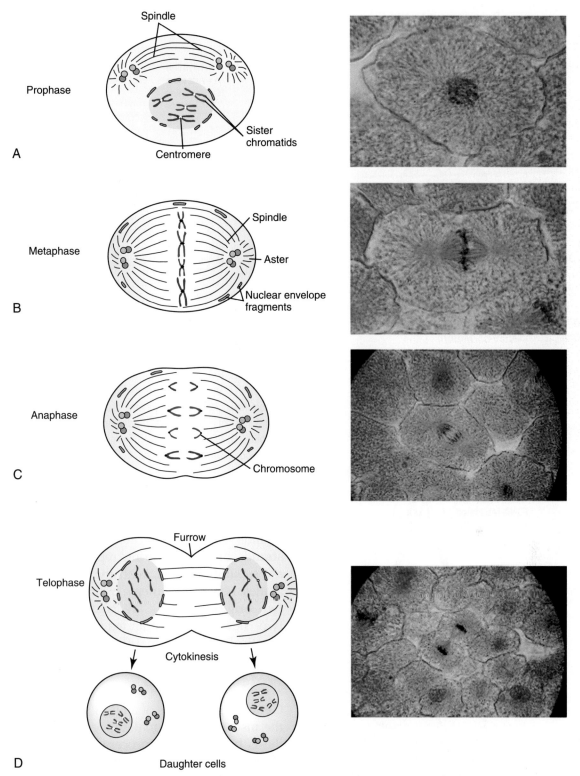

FIGURE 5.6 Mitosis. **A**, Prophase. **B**, Metaphase. **C**, Anaphase. **D**, Telophase. (Redrawn from VanMeter K, et al: *Microbiology for the healthcare professional*, St Louis, 2010, Mosby.)

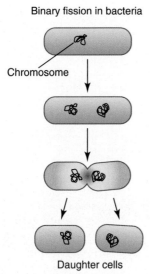

Binary fission in bacteria

Chromosome

Daughter cells

FIGURE 5.7 Binary fission. A single cell separates into two identical daughter cells, each with an identical copy of parent DNA. (Redrawn from VanMeter K, et al: *Microbiology for the healthcare professional*, St Louis, 2010, Mosby.)

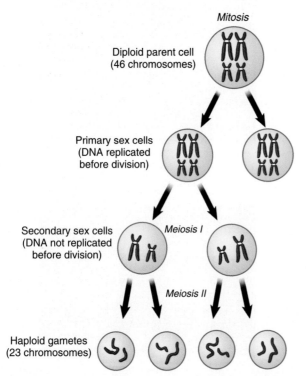

Mitosis

Diploid parent cell
(46 chromosomes)

Primary sex cells
(DNA replicated
before division)

Secondary sex cells
(DNA not replicated
before division)

Meiosis I

Meiosis II

Haploid gametes
(23 chromosomes)

FIGURE 5.8 Meiosis. Meiotic cell division takes place in two steps: *meiosis I* and *meiosis II*. Meiosis is called *reduction division* because the number of chromosomes is reduced by half (from the diploid number to the haploid number). (From Patton KT, Thibodeau GA: *Anatomy and physiology*, ed 9, St Louis, 2016, Mosby.)

Every DNA nucleotide contains one of four nitrogenous bases: adenine, thymine, guanine, and cytosine. Each base forms hydrogen bonds with another base on the complementary strand. The

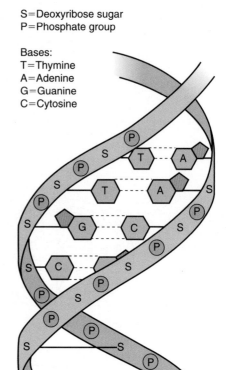

S=Deoxyribose sugar
P=Phosphate group

Bases:
T=Thymine
A=Adenine
G=Guanine
C=Cytosine

FIGURE 5.9 The DNA molecule. Representation of the DNA double helix showing the general structure of a nucleotide and the two kinds of "base pairs": adenine (A) with thymine (T) and guanine (G) with cytosine (C). (From Applegate: *The anatomy and physiology learning system*, ed 4, St Louis, 2011, Saunders.)

bases have a specific bonding pattern: adenine bonds with thymine, and guanine bonds with cytosine. Because of this method of bonding, the strands can be replicated, producing identical strands of DNA. During replication, the strands are separated. Then, with the help of several enzymes, new complementary strands for each of the two original strands are created. This produces two new double-stranded segments of DNA identical to the original (Fig. 5.10).

Protein Synthesis

Genes are segments of a DNA strand that provide the instructions for making proteins. Protein synthesis begins with a process called **transcription.** In this process, the genetic instructions on DNA are copied onto RNA strands called **messenger RNA (mRNA).** The mRNA strand has nitrogenous bases identical to those in DNA with the exception of uracil, which is substituted for thymine.

mRNA functions as a messenger that carries information from the original DNA helix in the nucleus to the ribosomes in the cytosol or on the rough ER. Here, the ribosome acts as the site of

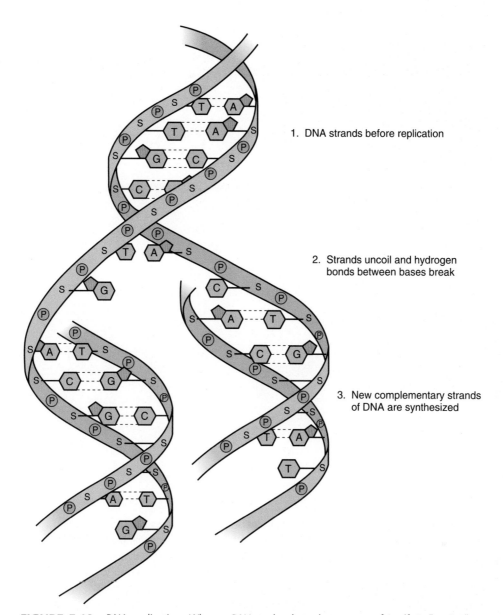

1. DNA strands before replication

2. Strands uncoil and hydrogen bonds between bases break

3. New complementary strands of DNA are synthesized

FIGURE 5.10 DNA replication. When a DNA molecule makes a copy of itself, it "unzips" to expose its nucleotide bases. Through the mechanism of obligatory base pairing, coordinated by the enzyme *DNA polymerase,* new DNA nucleotides bind to the exposed bases. This forms a new "other half" to each half of the original molecule. After all the bases have new nucleotides bound to them, two identical DNA molecules will be ready for distribution to the two daughter cells. (From Applegate: *The anatomy and physiology learning system,* ed 4, St Louis, 2011, Saunders.)

translation. Each group of three nucleotides along the stretch of mRNA is called a **codon,** and each of these codes for a specific **amino acid.** During translation, the ribosome moves forward along the mRNA strand, reading the information and assembling the amino acids in the correct sequence. The corresponding codon, or **anticodon,** is located on a unit called **transfer RNA (tRNA),** which carries a specific amino acid. tRNA molecules enter the ribosome and bind to specific mRNA codons to form a growing polypeptide (protein) chain. Eventually, the chain ends at what is called a **stop codon.** At this point, the chain is released into the cytoplasm and the protein folds onto itself and forms its complete conformation.

By dictating what is produced in translation through transcription, the DNA in the nucleus has control over everything taking place in the cell. The proteins that are produced will perform all the different cellular functions required for the cell's survival. The synthesis of proteins is summarized in Figure 5.11.

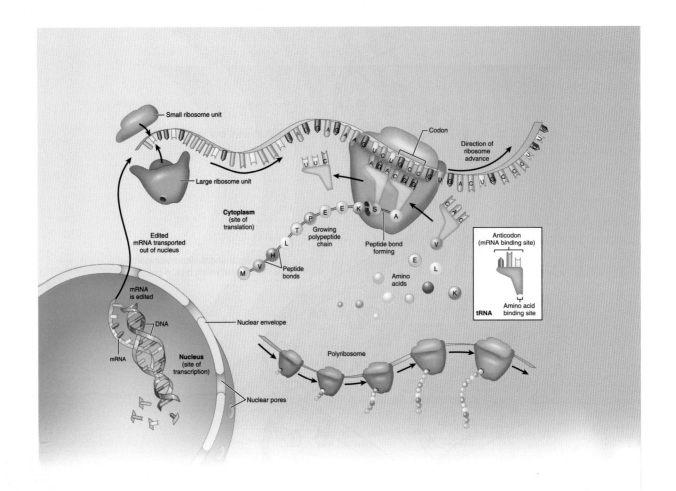

FIGURE 5.11 Protein synthesis begins with *transcription*, a process in which a messenger RNA (mRNA) molecule forms along one gene sequence of a DNA molecule within the cell's nucleus. As it is formed, the mRNA molecule separates from the DNA molecule, is edited, and leaves the nucleus through the large nuclear pores. Outside the nucleus, ribosome subunits attach to the beginning of the mRNA molecule and begin the process of *translation*. In translation, transfer RNA (tRNA) molecules bring specific amino acids—encoded by each mRNA codon—into place at the ribosome site. As the amino acids are brought into the proper sequence, they are joined together by peptide bonds to form long strands called *polypeptides*. Several polypeptide chains may be needed to make a complete protein molecule. (From Patton KT, Thibodeau GA: *Anatomy and physiology*, ed 9, St Louis, 2016, Mosby.)

Genetics

Genes are the basic units of heredity. Remember that a gene is a segment of a DNA molecule. Scientists have found that for every trait expressed in a sexually reproducing organism, there are at least two alternative versions of a gene called **alleles.** For simple traits, the versions can be one of two types: dominant or recessive. If both of the alleles are the same type, the organism is said to be **homozygous** for that trait. If they are different types, the organism is said to be **heterozygous.**

By using a device called a **Punnett square,** it is possible to predict genotype (the combination of alleles) and phenotype (what traits will be expressed) of the offspring of sexual reproduction.

Alleles are placed one per column for one gene and one per row for the other gene. In the example in Figure 5.12, a homozygous dominant is crossed with a heterozygous organism for the same trait. Note that all progeny will express dominance for this trait. In the example in Figure 5.13, three of the possible combinations will be dominant, and one will be recessive for this trait.

The Punnett square can be used to cross any number of different traits simultaneously. With these data, a probability of phenotypes that will be produced can be determined. However, the more traits desired, the more complex the cross.

Not all genes express themselves according to these simple rules, but they are the basis for all genetic understanding. There are many other methods of genetic expression. A few of these include multiple alleles, pleiotropy, epistasis, and polygenic inheritance.

HESI Hint

Because genetics is the study of heredity, many human disorders can be detected by studying a person's chromosomes or by creating a pedigree. A pedigree is a family tree that traces the occurrence of a certain trait through several generations. A pedigree is useful in understanding the genetic past as well as the possible future.

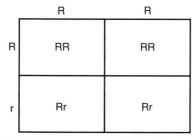

FIGURE 5.12 Punnett square depicting the cross between a homozygous dominant and a heterozygous organism.

	R	r
R	RR	Rr
r	Rr	rr

FIGURE 5.13 Punnett square depicting three possible dominant combinations.

Infectious Diseases

Germ theory is the currently accepted model of disease causation. Germ theory states that diseases are caused by living or nonliving microorganisms that invade a living host. Infectious diseases are spread by microorganisms such as bacteria, viruses, fungi, and protozoa.

Bacteria

Bacteria are single-celled prokaryotic microorganisms. Bacteria reproduce on their own and are able to survive inside and outside of the body. The two most common types of bacteria are rod-shaped *bacilli* and spherical *cocci*. Bacteria are also classified according to their cell wall structure, which is identified by *Gram staining*. Gram-positive bacteria have a cell wall composed primarily of a polysaccharide called peptidoglycan. The cell walls of Gram-negative bacteria have an extra lipid bilayer membrane outside the peptidoglycan layers, which makes them more resistant to antibiotics. Common bacterial infections include streptococcal pharyngitis (strep throat), *E. coli*, *C. difficile*, and Lyme disease.

HESI Hint

Gram Staining
A Gram stain is a crystal violet dye. When the dye is introduced to bacteria in a sample, the bacteria will either retain the violet/purple color or change color. Gram-positive bacteria retain the color of the dye. Gram-negative bacteria turn pink or red.

Viruses

Viruses are composed of genetic material (DNA or RNA) surrounded by a protein coat called a capsid. Viruses are smaller than bacteria, but unlike bacteria, viruses cannot survive without a host. Well-known viral infections include influenza, COVID-19, viral pneumonia, meningitis, and HIV.

Fungi

Fungi are spore-producing organisms that grow in the soil, on plants, in the water, and in the air. There are many thousands of species of fungi, but only a few pose a serious risk to humans. Some types of fungi cause infections on the skin and nails. Fungal spores in the air pose a greater risk of infection when they are inhaled into the lungs. Common types of pathogenic fungi are *Candida*, *Aspergillus*, and *Histoplasma*.

Protozoa

Protozoa are single-celled microorganisms that live in the water or in moist soil. Upon entering a human host, protozoa can multiply and cause serious disease. Infections caused by protozoa can spread through contaminated food or water, person-to-person contact, or vector transmission. Diseases caused by protozoa include malaria, giardia, amoebiasis, and trichomoniasis.

Chain of Infection

Infectious diseases spread when an infectious agent enters a susceptible host. The spread of infection is often described as a process involving six links that make up the **chain of infection** (Fig. 5.14). The first link in the chain is the infectious agent, or *pathogen*. Transmission occurs when the pathogen leaves its *reservoir* through a *portal of exit*, travels by a particular *mode of transmission*, and accesses a *portal of entry* to infect a *susceptible host*. A reservoir of infection is the place where a pathogen normally lives. Reservoirs include dirty surfaces, insects, animals, humans, and water. Portals of exit for a human reservoir include the respiratory tract, the gastrointestinal

tract, open wounds in the skin, or any potential pathway for blood or other fluids to exit the body. Modes of transmission are characterized as either direct or indirect (Box 5.1). Portals of entry often parallel the portal of exit; for example, respiratory secretions that exit a human reservoir by coughing or sneezing can enter another person through the nasal passages. The susceptible host is usually a person with a compromised immune system; this is why hospital-acquired infections are so common.

The Immune System

A healthy immune system can destroy pathogens before they cause disease. The immune system provides two levels of defense against invading pathogens. The first line of defense is the **innate immune system**. This system consists of physical barriers, which include the skin, body hair, and mucous membranes that line the lungs, gastrointestinal tract, and urinary tract. If a pathogen makes it past the physical barriers, the innate immune system produces an inflammatory response. White blood cells, or *leukocytes*, immediately travel to the area of infection and attack the pathogen. The host immune response begins with the arrival of white blood cells called phagocytes, which ingest and destroy invading cells. The two main types of phagocytes are neutrophils and macrophages. Neutrophils are the first immune cells to reach the site of infection, where they capture and destroy invading microorganisms and regulate the activity of macrophages. Other leukocytes involved in the immune response are basophils and mast cells, which release histamines that mediate the inflammatory response, and eosinophils, which mainly attack parasites that are too large to be destroyed by phagocytes.

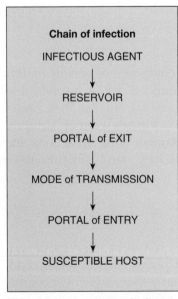

FIGURE 5.14 Chain of infection.

Box 5.1 Modes of Transmission

Direct Transmission
- Person-to-person contact
- Contact with body fluids
- Droplet spread

Indirect Transmission
- Airborne (respiratory particles)
- Vector-borne (organisms such as mosquitoes and ticks)
- Vehicle-borne (any nonliving object)

The **adaptive immune system** is the body's second line of defense, which is activated when the innate immune response fails to rid the body of infection. Adaptive immunity produces a response to a specific *antigen*. An antigen is a molecule on a pathogen that triggers an immune response in the host. The adaptive immune response is controlled by lymphocytes called B cells and T cells. B cells produce membrane-bound *antibodies*, which are proteins that bind to specific antigens. B cells circulate until all the antigens are removed from the body. This antibody-mediated response is called *humoral immunity*. T cells develop in the thymus gland and play a vital role in the adaptive immune system. Helper T cells identify specific antigens, but instead of binding with the antigen, they activate other immune cells (including B cells) to destroy the pathogen. Cytotoxic (killer) T cells recognize specific antigens and destroy the infected cells. The activation of cytotoxic T cells is called *cell-mediated immunity*. Once the infection is removed, some of the T and B cells become memory cells. T and B memory cells can recognize pathogens from a prior infection so the body can respond more quickly and prevent subsequent infection from occurring.

REVIEW QUESTIONS

1. Which is the smallest classification within the biological hierarchy?
   A. Family
   B. Order
   C. Genus
   D. Species

2. Which statement is true regarding the scientific process?
   A. A scientific experiment must be repeatable.
   B. All scientists must follow the exact same steps.
   C. The conclusion must support the hypothesis.
   D. The experiment is the final step of the process.

3. Which term represents the amount of heat necessary to raise the temperature of 1 gram of a substance by $1°C$?
   A. Specific heat
   B. Freezing point
   C. Boiling point
   D. Heat capacity

4. Which mechanism helps maintain homeostasis by reducing the effect of a stimulus?
   A. Anabolism
   B. Catabolism
   C. Negative feedback
   D. Positive feedback

5. The liver performs most of the body's detoxification. Which organelle(s) should you expect to be present in large amounts in liver cells?
   A. Rough endoplasmic reticulum
   B. Smooth endoplasmic reticulum
   C. Bound ribosomes
   D. Free ribosomes

6. What organelle converts food into energy for the cell?
   A. Lysosome
   B. Mitochondrion
   C. Nucleus
   D. Ribosome

7. Which equation describes aerobic respiration?
   A. Glucose + Oxygen → Carbon dioxide + Water
   B. Glucose → Lactate + Energy
   C. Glucose → Carbon dioxide + Energy
   D. Carbon dioxide + Water → Glucose + Oxygen

8. What are the end products of photosynthesis?
   A. Glucose and oxygen
   B. ATP and water
   C. NADH and oxygen
   D. Carbon dioxide and water

9. Which process occurs during interphase?
   A. Chromosomes align at the center of the cell.
   B. The nuclear envelope disappears.
   C. Chromosomes are duplicated.
   D. A parent cell separates into two daughter cells.

10. What is the name for an alternate version of a gene?
    A. Amino acid
    B. Codon
    C. Chromosome
    D. Allele

11. What is the end result of meiosis?
    A. Two haploid daughter cells
    B. Four haploid daughter cells
    C. Two diploid daughter cells
    D. Four diploid daughter cells
12. What sequence represents the process by which genetic instructions are delivered to the cell?
    A. Protein → DNA → RNA
    B. DNA → RNA → protein
    C. RNA → DNA → protein
    D. Protein → RNA → DNA
13. What is the first step of protein synthesis?
    A. Instructions in the DNA are copied onto mRNA.
    B. mRNA binds with ribosomes in the cytoplasm.
    C. tRNA carries amino acids to the ribosomal binding sites.
    D. Anticodons bind with complementary codons to form a base pair.
14. What bacterial characteristic is determined by Gram staining?
    A. Size
    B. Shape
    C. Cell wall structure
    D. Reproductive method
15. What type of white blood cell produces antibodies?
    A. Lymphocytes
    B. Basophils
    C. Eosinophils
    D. Neutrophils

ANSWERS TO REVIEW QUESTIONS

1. D
2. A
3. A
4. C
5. B
6. B
7. A
8. A
9. C
10. D
11. B
12. B
13. A
14. C
15. A

CHEMISTRY

Chemistry is a part of our everyday lives. Almost three quarters of the objective information in a client's medical record consists of laboratory data derived from chemical analytical testing. Laboratory tests and chemical analysis play an important role in the detection, identification, and management of most diseases. The client's evaluation, diagnosis, treatment, care, and prognosis are, at least in part, based on the chemical information from laboratory tests that involve traditional technologies of chemistry. A sound, basic knowledge of chemistry enables the healthcare professional to reduce the risk of mishandled biologic samples and misdiagnosis, and thereby deliver safer and higher quality care.

Chemistry is the study of matter and its properties. Everything in the universe is made or composed of different kinds of matter in one of its three states: solid, liquid, or gas. Matter is defined by its properties, and chemistry is a study of those properties and how those properties relate to one another. Chemistry is a very broad field of study and can be divided into many areas of specialization, such as physical or general chemistry, biochemistry, and organic and inorganic chemistry. This chapter reviews chemistry from the most basic of substances to very complex compounds.

CHAPTER OUTLINE

KEY TERMS

Acid
Alloy
Amalgam
Atom
Atomic Number
Atomic Weight
Base
Basic Unit of Measure
Biochemistry
Catalysts
Celsius
Chemical Equations

Combustion
Compound
Covalent Bond
Decomposition
Deoxyribose
Double Replacement
Electron
Electron Clouds
Equilibrium
Fahrenheit
Gas-gas solutions
Groups

Ionic Bond
Isotopes
Kelvin
Mass Number
Mathematical Sign
Mole
Neutron
Nucleus
Orbit
Periodic Table
Periods
pH

Scientific Notation, The Metric System, and Temperature Scales

Scientific Notation

Scientific notation is the scientific system of writing numbers. Scientific notation is a method to write very big or very small numbers easily. Scientific notation is composed of three parts: a **mathematical sign** (+ or −), the **significand**, and the exponential, sometimes called the *logarithm*.

1. The mathematical sign designates whether the number is positive or negative.

> **HESI Hint**
>
> There is an understood (+) before a positive significand as there is in all positive numbers.

2. The significand is the base value of the number or the value of the number when all the values of ten are removed.
3. The exponential is a multiplier of the significand in powers of ten (Table 6.1). A positive exponential multiplies the significand by factors of ten. A negative exponential multiplies the significand by factors of one tenth (0.1).

Table 6.1 Exponentials

10^9	1,000,000,000
10^6	1,000,000
10^3	1,000
10^2	100
10^1	10
10^0	1
10^{-2}	0.01
10^{-6}	0.000001
10^{-9}	0.000000001

*1.0 is understood to be the significand with each of the above exponentials.

> **HESI Hint**
>
> Some calculators or other devices may write the exponent as an "e" or "E" as in 3.2 e5 or 3.2 E5, called E notation, instead of 3.2×10^5, but it means the same.

Example

Consider -9.0462×10^5, where the minus (−) sign makes this a negative number, 9.0462 is the significand or base value, and 10^5 is the exponential or multiplier of the significand in the power of 10. In the example above, -9.0462×10^5 equals $-9.0462 \times 10 \times 10 \times 10 \times 10 \times 10$ or −904,620.

Example

Consider 4.7×10^{-3}, where the absence of the (+) sign is understood as positive, 4.7 is the significand or base value, and 10^{-3} is the exponential or multiplier of the significand in the negative power of ten (as tenths). In the example above, 4.7×10^{-3} equals $(4.7 \times 0.1 \times 0.1 \times 0.1)$ or 0.0047.

> **HESI Hint**
>
> Move the decimal in the significand the number of places equal to the exponent of 10. When the exponent is positive, the number is a large value. For example: 3.4×10^5 m = 340,000 m. When the exponent is negative, the number is a value smaller than 1. For example: 2.9×10^{-3} L = 0.0029 L.

> **HESI Hint**
>
> When writing a number between −1 and +1, always place a zero (0) to the left of the decimal. Write 0.62 and −0.39 (do not write .62 or −.39) to avoid mistakes when reading the number and locating the decimal.

The Metric System of Measurement

The metric system is a method to measure weight, length, and volume. It is a simple, logical, and efficient measurement system that is the standard in health professions. The basic measurements of the metric system are grams, liters, and meters. A gram (g) is the basic measure of weight, a liter (L) is the basic measure of volume, and a meter (m) is the basic measure of distance.

Each metric measurement is composed of a metric prefix and a basic unit of measure. An example is "kilogram," where "kilo" is the **prefix** and "gram" is the **basic unit of measure**. The prefixes have the same meaning or value, regardless of which basic unit of measurement (grams, liters, or meters) is used. Prefixes are the quantifiers of the measurement units. All of the prefixes are based on multiples of ten. Any *one* of the prefixes can be combined with *one* of the basic units of measurement. Some examples are deciliter (dL), kilogram (kg), and millimeter (mm) (Table 6.2).

HESI Hint

Some comparisons may give more insight into sizes or amounts. A meter is a little more than 3 inches longer than a yard. A dime is a little less than 2 cm in diameter. A kilogram is about 2.2 lb. A liter is a little more than a quart.

Temperature Scales

The three most common temperature systems are **Fahrenheit**, **Celsius**, and **Kelvin**.

Fahrenheit (F) is a temperature measuring system used only in the United States, its territories, Belize, and Jamaica. It is rarely used for any scientific measurements except for body temperature (see Table 6.3). It has the following characteristics:

- Zero degrees (0°F) is the freezing point of sea water or heavy brine at sea level.
- 32°F is the freezing point of pure water at sea level.
- 212°F is the boiling point of pure water at sea level.
- Most people have a body temperature of 98.6°F.

Celsius (sometimes called Centigrade) is a temperature system used in the rest of the world and by the scientific community. It has the following characteristics:

- Zero degrees (0°C) is the freezing point of pure water at sea level.
- 100°C is the boiling point of pure water at sea level.
- Most people have a body temperature of 37°C.

Table 6.3 Important Temperatures in Fahrenheit and Celsius

Condition	EXAMPLES OF CELSIUS (C) AND FAHRENHEIT (F) TEMPERATURES	
Freezing water	0°C	32°F
Normal body temperature	37°C	98.6°F
Boiling water	100°C	212°F

Table 6.2 The Prefixes

Prefix	Abbreviation	Means	Numerically
Tera	T-	10^{12}	1 trillion times
Giga	G-	10^9	1 billion times
Mega	M-	10^6	1 million times
Kilo	k-	10^3	1 thousand times
Hecto	h-	10^2	1 hundred times
Deka	D-	10^1	10 times
Deci	d-	10^{-1}	1 tenth of
Centi	c-	10^{-2}	1 hundredth of
Milli	m-	10^{-3}	1 thousandth of
Micro	μ-	10^{-6}	1 millionth of
Nano	n-	10^{-9}	1 billionth of
Pico	p-	10^{-12}	1 trillionth of
Femto	f-	10^{-15}	1 quadrillionth of

Kelvin (K) is used only in the scientific community. Kelvin has the following characteristics:

- Zero Kelvin (0K) is −273.15°C and is thought to be the lowest temperature achievable or absolute zero (0).
- The freezing point of water is 273K.
- The boiling point of water is 373K.
- Most people have a body temperature of 310K, but this is never used.

Atomic Structure and the Periodic Table

Atomic Structure

The basic building block of all molecules is the **atom.** An atom's physical structure is that of a **nucleus** and **orbits**, sometimes called **electron clouds.** The nucleus is at the center of the atom and is composed of **protons** and **neutrons.** At the outermost part of the atom are the orbits of the **electrons**, which spin around the nucleus at fantastic speeds, forming electron clouds. The speed of the electrons is so great that, in essence, they occupy the space around the nucleus as a cloud rather than as discrete individual locations. The electrons orbit the nucleus at various energy levels called *shells* or *orbits*, almost like the layers of an onion. As each orbital is filled to capacity, atoms begin adding electrons to the next orbit. An atom is most stable when its outermost orbit is full. However, most of the volume of an atom is empty space. See Fig. 6.1 for examples of atoms.

Protons have a positive electrical charge, electrons have a negative charge, and neutrons have no charge at all. Ground state atoms tend to have equal numbers of protons and electrons, making them electrically neutral. When an atom is electrically charged, it is called an *ion* or it is said to be in an ionic state. This usually occurs when it is in a solution or in the form of a chemical compound. An atom in an ionic state will have lost electrons, resulting in a net positive charge, or will have gained electrons, resulting in a net negative charge. The atom is called a *cation* if it has a positive charge and an *anion* if it has a negative charge.

The Periodic Table

Matter is defined by its properties. It can also be stated that the properties of matter come from the properties of its composite elements, and the periodic table organizes the elements based on their structure and thus helps predict the properties of each of the elements (Fig. 6.2).

The **periodic table** is made up of a series of rows called **periods** (hence the name periodic table) and columns called **groups**. It is, at its simplest, a table of the known elements arranged according to their properties. The periodic table makes it possible to predict, for example, the charge of an atom or element, when it exists as an ion, by its location in the table. Group IA has a plus one (+1) charge, group IIA has a positive two (+2) charge, and group IIIA has a positive three (+3) charge. Group IVA can have either a positive four (+4) or a negative four (−4) charge. The negative charges are as follows: group VA has a negative three (−3) charge, group VIA has a negative two (−2) charge, and group VIIA has a negative one (−1) charge. Group VIIIA, called the noble gases, has no charge when in solution; it remains neutral in nearly all situations. Another property that can be generally deduced by the periodic chart is the number of electrons in the outer electron shell or cloud. Group IA will have one (1) electron in its outer shell. Group IIA will have two (2), Group IIIA will have three (3), Group IVA will have four (4), and on through all the A groups. Groups 3 IIIB through 12 IIB are called *transition metals* and are not as straightforward to predict because of some exceptions to the rules.

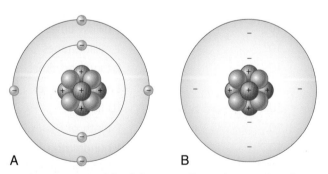

A   B

FIGURE 6.1   Models of the atom. The nucleus consists of protons (+) and neutrons at the core. Electrons inhabit outer regions called **(A)** electron shells or energy levels or **(B)** clouds. (From Patton KT, Thibodeau GA: *Anatomy and physiology*, ed 9, St Louis, 2016, Mosby.)

HESI Hint

An important principle to remember is that the properties of each element can be predicted based on its location in the periodic chart.

Periodic table legend:
- ▣ Major elements
- ☐ Trace elements

Example cell:
- 6 — Atomic number (number of protons)
- C — Chemical symbol
- 12.011 — Atomic weight (number of protons plus average number of neutrons)

1 H 1.008																	2 He 4.002
3 Li 6.941	4 Be 9.012											5 B 10.811	6 C 12.011	7 N 14.007	8 O 15.999	9 F 18.998	10 Ne 20.180
11 Na 22.990	12 Mg 24.305											13 Al 26.982	14 Si 28.086	15 P 30.974	16 S 32.066	17 Cl 35.452	18 Ar 39.948
19 K 39.098	20 Ca 40.078	21 Sc 44.956	22 Ti 47.867	23 V 50.942	24 Cr 51.996	25 Mn 54.931	26 Fe 55.845	27 Co 58.933	28 Ni 58.963	29 Cu 63.546	30 Zn 65.39	31 Ga 69.723	32 Ge 72.61	33 As 74.922	34 Se 78.96	35 Br 79.904	36 Kr 83.80
37 Rb 85.468	38 Sr 87.62	39 Y 88.906	40 Zr 91.224	41 Nb 92.906	42 Mo 95.94	43 Tc (98)	44 Ru 101.07	45 Rh 102.906	46 Pd 106.42	47 Ag 107.868	48 Cd 112.411	49 In 114.818	50 Sn 118.710	51 Sb 121.760	52 Te 127.60	53 I 126.904	54 Xe 131.29
55 Cs 132.905	56 Ba 137.327	57 La 138.905	72 Hf 178.49	73 Ta 180.948	74 W 183.84	75 Re 186.207	76 Os 190.23	77 Ir 192.217	78 Pt 195.08	79 Au 196.967	80 Hg 200.59	81 Ti 204.383	82 Pb 207.2	83 Bi 208.980	84 Po (209)	85 At (210)	86 Rn (222)
87 Fr (223)	88 Ra 226.025	89 Ac 227.028	104 Rf (263.113)	105 Db (262.114)	106 Sg (266.122)	107 Bh (264.125)	108 Hs (269.134)	109 Mt (268.139)	110 Ds (272.146)	111 Rg (272.154)	112 Uub (277)	113 Uut (284)	114 Uuq (289)	115 Uup (288)	116 Uuh (292)	117 Uus (292)	118 Uuo (294)

58 Ce 140.115	59 Pr 140.907	60 Nd 144.24	61 Pm (145)	62 Sm 150.36	63 Eu 151.965	64 Eu 157.25	65 Gd 158.925	66 Tb 162.50	67 Ho 164.930	68 Er 167.26	69 Tm 168.939	70 Yb 173.04	71 Lu 174.967
90 Th 232.038	91 Pa 231.036	92 U 238.029	93 Np 237.048	94 Pu (244)	95 Am (243)	96 Cm (247)	97 Bk (247)	98 Cf (251)	99 Es (252)	100 Fm (257)	101 Md (258)	102 No (259)	103 Lr (260)

FIGURE 6.2 Periodic table of elements. (From Patton KT, Thibodeau GA: *Anatomy and physiology*, ed 9, St Louis, 2016, Mosby.)

Atomic Number and Atomic Weight

Two important numbers or properties of atoms that can be obtained from the periodic table are the atomic number and the atomic mass.

The **atomic number** is the number of protons in the nucleus, and it defines an atom as a particular element. For instance, any atom that has eleven (11) protons, no matter how many neutrons or electrons, is sodium (Na). If an atom has six (6) protons, it is carbon (C). The atomic number is located at the top of each of the squares in a periodic table. It is always a whole number.

The **atomic weight** of an atom is the *average* mass of each of that element's **isotopes**. Isotopes are different kinds of the same atom that vary in weight. Protons and neutrons each have approximately the same mass or weight, which makes up nearly all of the atom's total mass. The atomic weight is the number at the bottom of each of the squares in the periodic table, and it is usually a decimal number. For a given element, the number of protons remains the same, whereas the number of neutrons varies to make the different isotopes. The combined number of protons and neutrons of an element is the **mass number** (which is not listed on the periodic table). The most common isotope of small atoms, generally, has the same number of protons and neutrons in its nucleus. The element

Carbon 12 (^{12}C), the most common carbon, has six (6) protons and six (6) neutrons. The isotope used for "carbon dating" is Carbon 14 (^{14}C), which has six (6) protons and eight (8) neutrons.

HESI Hint

The terms atomic weight and **atomic mass** are often used interchangeably, but they are not the same. Atomic mass is the mass of a *single atom*, whereas atomic weight is the weighted average of an atom and its isotopes. Atomic mass is *approximately* equal to mass number but is slightly larger because it takes into account all subatomic particles that contribute to the mass of an atom.

Chemical Equations

An element or atom is the simplest form of matter that can naturally exist in nature. It can exist as a pure element or in combination with other elements. When they exist in combination with other elements, the combination is called a **compound**, and they combine in whole number ratios. A part of an element does not naturally exist; at least one atom of the element is present in a chemical reaction. For instance, the elements sodium (Na) and chlorine (Cl) will combine perfectly as whole elements or atoms in a one-to-one ratio to make the compound table salt (NaCl).

Chemical equations are simply recipes. Ingredients, called **reactants**, react to produce desired end results or compounds called **products**. Equations are written in the following manner:

Reactants → Products

In any chemical reaction, an arrow between the reactants and the products is present. This arrow symbolizes the direction of the reaction. Some reactions move toward the product side as seen above, and some reactions will move toward the reactant side with an arrow pointing toward the reactants instead of the products.

Reactants ← Products

There are also reactions that will create both reactants and products at the same time.

Reactants ↔ Products

An example is the reaction of aqueous silver nitrate ($AgNO_3$) and aqueous potassium chloride (KCl) to produce solid silver chloride (AgCl) and potassium nitrate (KNO_3).

$$AgNO_3 + KCl \rightarrow AgCl + KNO_3$$

Silver nitrate + potassium chloride yields

Silver chloride + potassium nitrate

The law of conservation of mass states that mass cannot be created or destroyed during a chemical reaction. Therefore, once the reactants have been written and the products predicted, the equation must be balanced. The same number of each element must be represented on both sides of the equation. The above example has one silver atom, one nitrogen atom, three oxygen atoms, one potassium atom, and one chloride atom on each side of the equation. Therefore, nothing in the way of matter was created or destroyed; it was simply rearranged.

Equilibrium and Reversibility

A chemical reaction may proceed to completion, but some reactions may stop before all of the reactants are used to make products. These reactions are said to be at **equilibrium**. Equilibrium is a state in which reactants are forming products at the same rate that products are forming reactants. A reaction at equilibrium can be said to be reversible. As the chemicals A and B react to create

C and D, C and D react to make more A and B at the same rate.

$$A + B \leftrightarrow C + D$$

Through manipulation of the reaction by various means, shifts in equilibrium reversibility or the rate of the reaction can be controlled.

Reaction Rates

Chemical reactions generally proceed at a specific rate. Some reactions are fast, and some are slow. There are basically four ways to increase the reaction rate: increase the temperature in the reaction, increase the surface area of the reactants, add a catalyst, or increase the concentrations of reactants.

Increasing the Temperature

Increasing the temperature causes the particles to have a greater kinetic energy, thereby causing them to move around faster, increasing their chances of contact and the energy with which they collide. Collisions are necessary for the chemical reactions to occur.

Increasing the Surface Area

Increasing the surface area of the particles in the reaction gives the particles more opportunity to come into contact with one another. Wood shavings are an excellent example. One can increase the surface area of a log by cutting it into shavings or sawdust. Wood in the form of sawdust will burn or react much faster than a whole log.

Catalysts

A **catalyst** accelerates a reaction by reducing the activation energy or the amount of energy necessary for a reaction to occur. The catalyst is not used up in the reaction and can be collected at completion of the reaction. Various substances can be catalysts. Common examples include metals and proteins (protein catalysts are called enzymes).

Increasing the Concentration

Increasing the concentration of the reactants will cause more chance collisions between the reactants and produce more products. By analogy, if there are more cars on the road, there are likely to be more accidents or collisions. The more reactants there are, the faster and more often they will bump into each other and react or become products.

Solutions and Solution Concentrations

Solutions

A **solution** can be defined as a homogeneous mixture of two or more substances. In a solution, there is one or more **solute(s)**, the part or parts that are being dissolved, and the **solvent**, the part that is doing the dissolving. Simple solutions are common in the lab and contain one solute mixed into the solvent, like pure sodium chloride dissolved in pure water. Complex solutions are more commonly found in everyday life and contain multiple solutes mixed into the solvent. Carbonated beverages are an example of a complex solution with many compounds including colorants, flavoring, carbon dioxide gas, and sugar that are mixed into water to form the solution. Solutions can be a liquid in a liquid, a solid in a liquid, or a solid in a solid. The following are types of solutions:

- **Alloys:** Solid solutions of metals to make a new one such as bronze, which is copper and tin, or steel, which is iron and carbon, and may contain tungsten, chromium, and manganese.
- **Amalgams:** A specific type of alloy in which a metal is dissolved in mercury.
- **Gas-gas solutions:** Air is a solution of gases that contains O_2, CO_2, and Ar as solutes, and N_2 as the solvent.

Concentration of Solutions—Percent Concentration

Concentration is expressed as weight per weight, as in grams per grams; weight per volume, as in grams per liters; or volume per volume, as in milliliters per liter. Percent concentration is the expression of concentrations as parts per 100 parts. Therefore, most concentrations of this type are expressed as milligrams (mg) per 100 milliliters (mL), which can also be written as mg/100mL or mg/dL. This is commonly used for solids like NaCl dissolved in water: 12 mg NaCl/100 mL solution. A concentration expression of milliliters (mL) per 100 milliliters (mL) can be written as mL/100mL or mL/dL. This is commonly used for liquid-liquid mixtures: 4.3 mL alcohol/100 mL of solution.

Concentration of Solutions—Molar Concentration

Molarity, or molar concentration, is a more sophisticated way to express concentrations than percent. One of the most important concepts in chemistry is the "mole." A **mole** is 6.02×10^{23} molecules of something. This number, 6.02×10^{23}, which is more than a trillion trillions, is known as *Avogadro's number*. A one molar solution will contain 6.02×10^{23} representative molecules of a solute in a liter of solvent. Molar concentrations are written as mol/L. It is important to note that if the atomic mass of any element is measured in grams (g), then one mole or 6.02×10^{23} atoms of that element or compound will have been weighed out.

Chemical Reactions

A chemical reaction involves making or changing chemical bonds between elements or compounds to create new chemical compounds with different chemical formulas and different chemical properties. There are five main types of chemical reactions: synthesis, decomposition, combustion, single replacement, and double replacement. When a reaction occurs, the product is generally a molecule. A molecule may have a subscript written after the chemical symbol as in O_2, which is oxygen.

In a **synthesis** reaction, two elements combine to form a product. An example is the formation of ammonia when the element nitrogen reacts with hydrogen:

$$N_2 + 3H_2 \rightarrow 2NH_3$$

One nitrogen + three hydrogens yields two ammonia molecules.

Decomposition is often described as the opposite of synthesis because it is the breaking of a compound into parts.

$$2KClO_3 \rightarrow 2KCl + 3O_2$$

When heated, the solid potassium chlorate breaks down into solid potassium chloride and oxygen gas.

Combustion is a self-sustaining, exothermic (creates heat) chemical reaction where oxygen and a fuel compound such as a hydrocarbon react. In the combustion of hydrocarbon (gas or oil product), the products are carbon dioxide (CO_2) and water (H_2O). The combustion of ethane (C_2H_6)

would look like this in a chemical equation, where (g) stands for gas:

$$2C_2H_6 \ (g) + 7O_2 \ (g) \ \rightarrow 4CO_2 \ (g) + 6H_2O \ (g)$$

Replacement reactions involve ionic compounds; whether or not the reaction will take place is based on the reactivity of the metals involved. **Single replacement** reactions consist of a more active metal reacting with an ionic compound containing a less active metal to produce a new compound. A good example is the reaction of copper (Cu) with aqueous silver nitrate ($AgNO_3$). The copper (Cu) and the silver (Ag) simply swap places. This type of reaction is referred to as single replacement and is illustrated in the following equation, where (aq) stands for aqueous and (s) stands for solid:

$$Cu \ (s) + 2AgNO_3 \ (aq) \ \rightarrow Cu(NO_3)_2 \ (aq) + 2Ag \ (s)$$

Copper + silver nitrate yields

copper nitrate + silver

Double replacement reactions involve two ionic compounds. The positive ion from one compound combines with the negative ion of the other compound. The result is two new ionic compounds that have "switched partners." The example of the reaction of silver nitrate ($AgNO_3$) and potassium chloride (KCl) is a good representation of double replacement:

$$AgNO_3 + KCl \ \rightarrow \ AgCl + KNO_3$$

Silver nitrate + potassium chloride yields
silver chloride + potassium nitrate

Chemical Bonding

Chemical bonding is the joining of one atom, element, or chemical to another. Some bonds are very weak, and some are nearly unbreakable. In many cases the type of bonding will be determined by the interplay of the electrons in the outer shell of the atom. There are two main types of chemical bonding: ionic and covalent.

An **ionic bond** is an electrostatic attraction between two oppositely charged ions, or a cation and an anion. This type of bond is generally formed between a metal and a nonmetal. An excellent example of ionic bonding is salt. Since opposites attract, the positive cation will attract the negative anion and form an electrostatic bond. Sodium (Na) becomes positively charged when it loses the

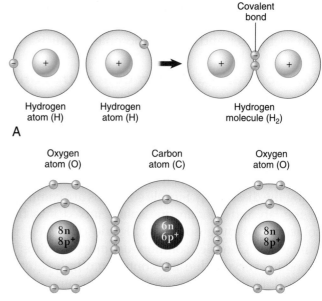

FIGURE 6.3 Types of covalent bonds. **A,** A single covalent bond forms by the sharing of one electron pair between two atoms of hydrogen, resulting in a molecule of hydrogen gas. **B,** A double covalent bond (double bond) forms by the sharing of two pairs of electrons between two atoms. In this case, two double bonds form: one between carbon and each of the two oxygen atoms. (From Patton KT, Thibodeau GA: *Anatomy and physiology,* ed 9, St Louis, 2016, Mosby.)

outermost electron to become a cation (Na^+). Chlorine (Cl) becomes negatively charged when it gains an electron to become an anion (Cl^-). Then, the compound is formed when the cation and anion attract to form a neutral compound.

$$Na^+ + Cl^- \ \rightarrow \ NaCl$$

Sodium ion + chloride ion yields (table) salt

A **covalent bond** is formed when two atoms *share* electrons, generally in pairs, with one pair from each atom. A single covalent bond is the sharing of one pair of electrons. A double covalent bond is formed when two electron pairs are shared, and a triple covalent bond is formed when three electron pairs are shared. The covalent bond is the strongest of any type of chemical bond and is generally formed between two nonmetals (Fig. 6.3).

In a covalently bonded compound, if the electrons in the bond are shared equally, the bond is termed *nonpolar.* However, not all elements share electrons equally within a bond. When this occurs, a polar bond is the result, which means that the shared electron density of the bond is concentrated around one atom more than the other. Polarity is based on the difference in electronegativity values for the elements involved in the bond. The greater the difference, the more polar the bond will be, or one end or side of the molecule will have a charge distinctly more positive and the other side of the molecule will be more negative in charge, forming what is a called a dipole.

There are other types of attractions between particles called *intermolecular forces*. These are not bonding interactions between atoms within a molecule but instead are weaker forces of attraction between whole molecules. These forces are hydrogen bonding, dipole-dipole interactions, and dispersion forces.

A *hydrogen bond* is the attraction for a hydrogen atom by a highly electronegative element. The elements generally involved are fluorine (F), oxygen (O), and nitrogen (N). Hydrogen bonds are about 5%–10% as strong as covalent bonds, making them the strongest of the intermolecular forces.

A *dipole-dipole interaction* is the attraction of one dipole on one molecule for the dipole of another molecule. A dipole is created when an electron pair is shared unequally in a covalent bond between two atoms or elements (discussed earlier in polar covalent bonding). Because the electrons are shared unequally, the molecule, not the covalent bond, will have a positive end and a negative end or side. In a solution, the molecules will align the charged ends of the molecule north to south or positive to negative, where the north end on one molecule is next to the south end of another. The result is a weak bond between molecules, where the more highly electropositive end of a molecule is attracted to the electronegative end of another molecule. This attraction is considered a weak intermolecular force. It is only about 1% as strong as a normal covalent bond.

Dispersion forces, sometimes called London dispersion forces, are the weakest of all the intermolecular forces. Sometimes the electrons within an element or compound will concentrate themselves on one side of an atom. This causes a momentary or temporary dipole, which would be attracted to another momentary dipole of opposite charge in another near element or compound.

Stoichiometry

Stoichiometry is the part of chemistry that deals with the quantities and numeric relationships of the participants in a chemical reaction. For a chemical equation to be balanced, numbers called coefficients are placed in front of each compound. These numbers are used in a ratio to compare how much of one substance is needed to react with another in a certain reaction. The process is similar to comparing ingredients in a recipe.

$$2C_2H_6 + 7O_2 \rightarrow 4CO_2 + 6H_2O$$

Ethane + oxygen yields carbon dioxide + water

Using this reaction, determine the number of moles of oxygen (O_2) that will react with four (4) moles of ethane (C_2H_6). It is possible to determine the number of moles of oxygen needed to complete the reaction using a process called *dimensional analysis*:

$$\frac{4 \text{ mol } C_2H_6}{} \left| \frac{7 \text{ mol } O_2}{2 \text{ mol } C_2H_6} \right. = 14 \text{ mol } O_2$$

By multiplying the given amount of four moles of ethane by the actual amount of seven moles of oxygen (O_2) and dividing by the actual number of two moles of ethane (C_2H_6), one can determine that the number of moles of oxygen needed to react will be fourteen (14).

Oxidation and Reduction

Oxidation/reduction reactions, called *redox*, involve the transfer of electrons from one element to another. *Oxidation is the loss of electrons, and reduction is the gain of electrons.* It is not possible to have one without the other. The element that is oxidized (loses electron) is the reductant or reducing agent, and the element that is reduced (gains electron) is the oxidant or the oxidizing agent. Even though a substance is oxidized and gains an electron, its ionic charge is more negative; likewise a substance that is reduced loses an electron, and its ionic charge is more positive.

HESI Hint

A good mnemonic is "OIL-RIG" or Oxidation Is Loss (of an electron), Reduction Is Gain (of an electron). Think of it this way: to "reduce" an element, one must cause that element's overall electrical charge to become less, and that is done by adding or gaining one or more negatively charged electrons (e^-).

A Redox Reaction

$$\underset{\text{Reduced}}{\text{Oxidant (gains electron)} + e^-} \leftrightarrow \underset{\text{Oxidized}}{\text{Reductant (loses electron)} - e^-}$$

The oxidant is reduced because it gains an electron. The reductant is oxidized because it loses an electron.

To identify what has been oxidized and what has been reduced, the oxidation states of all elements in the compound must be determined. The following is a series of rules to make those determinations:

1. The oxidation number of any elemental atom is zero. This means that if an element is in its *natural* state, its charge or number is zero. Most elements in their standard states are single atoms. However, a few exceptions exist including hydrogen (H_2), bromine (Br_2), oxygen (O_2), nitrogen (N_2), iodine (I_2), fluorine (F_2), and chlorine (Cl_2). When these elements exist outside of a compound in their natural state, they are always in pairs.
2. The oxidation number of any simple ion is the charge of the ion. If in a reaction, sodium (Na) was listed as an ion (Na^+), it would have an oxidation number of plus one ($+1$). If chlorine (Cl) was listed as an ion (Cl^-), it would have an oxidation number of minus one (-1).
3. The oxidation number for oxygen in a compound is minus two (-2).
4. The oxidation number for hydrogen in a compound is plus one ($+1$).
5. The sum of the oxidation numbers equals the charge on the molecules or polyatomic ions.

Example: Assign oxidation numbers to all elements in the following reactions:

$$2C_2H_6 + 7O_2 \rightarrow 4CO_2 + 6H_2O$$

Ethane + oxygen yields carbon dioxide + water

By using the rules listed earlier, we can use simple algebra to solve for the change of electrical charges of those elements not discussed in the rules. In solving for carbon, the first element in the first reactant, ethane (C_2H_6), we can ignore the coefficient because it has nothing to do with the oxidation states of any of the elements. The total charge on the compound is zero, as is determined using rule five. From rule four, hydrogen must have an oxidation state of $+1$. There are six hydrogen molecules, so the total charge of the

hydrogen molecules is $+6$. Following is the algebra to solve for the oxidation state of carbon (x):

$$2x + 6(+1) = 0$$

Solving for x, carbon is found to have a charge of -3.

If the same method is used, the states of all the other elements can be determined. Oxygen in O_2 is zero (rule one). Carbon in CO_2 is $+4$, and oxygen is -2. Finally, hydrogen in water is $+1$, and oxygen is -2. With this information, it is possible to predict what is oxidized and what is reduced. Look at the charges on either side of the equation and see what has changed. Carbon goes from a state of -3 to a state of $+4$. It has lost seven electrons and has, therefore, been oxidized. Oxygen's state has changed from 0 to -2. It has gained two electrons and has, therefore, been reduced.

Acids and Bases

Acids are corrosive to metals; they change blue litmus paper red and become less acidic when mixed with bases. **Bases**, also called *alkaline compounds*, are substances that denature proteins, making them feel very slick; they change red litmus paper blue and become less basic when mixed with acids.

Acids are compounds that are hydrogen or proton donors. *Hydrogen in its ionic state is simply a proton.* In water, unattached protons exist only for a short time before reacting with other water molecules to produce H_3O^+, a substance called hydronium. Hydronium is a water molecule plus a proton or hydrogen.

Bases are hydrogen or proton acceptors and generally have a hydroxide (OH) group in the makeup of the molecule. This definition explains the dissociation of water into low concentrations of hydronium and hydroxide ions:

$$H_2O + H_2O \leftrightarrow H_3O^+ + OH^-$$

Water + water yields acid + base

In this example, one water (H_2O) molecule acts as a hydrogen donor, giving one of its two hydrogens to another water molecule and in the process producing the hydronium (H_3O^+) cation and leaving a hydroxyl group (OH^-). All acids produce hydronium when placed in H_2O. As can be seen, H_2O is amphoteric, which means it can act as both an acid and a base. In the example above, one molecule of H_2O acts as the proton donor, becoming a hydroxide (OH), and another molecule acts as the proton acceptor, becoming the conjugate acid (H_3O^+).

The concentration of acids is expressed as **pH.** The pH scale commonly in use ranges from 0 to 14 and is a measure of the acidity or alkalinity of a solution (Fig. 6.4). A neutral solution that is neither acidic nor basic has a value of 7. Lower numbers mean more acidic, and higher numbers mean more basic.

Nuclear Chemistry

Chemical and nuclear reactions are quite different. In chemical reactions, atoms react to reach stable electron configurations. Nuclear chemistry is concerned with reactions that take place in the

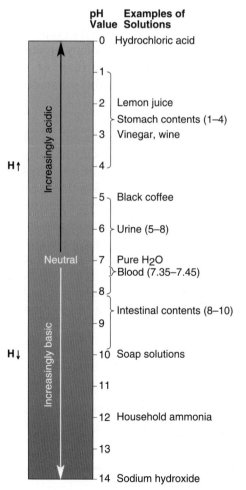

FIGURE 6.4 The pH range. (From Herlihy B: *The human body in health and illness*, ed 5, St Louis, 2014, Saunders.)

nucleus to obtain stable nuclear configurations. *Radioactivity* is the word used to describe the emission of particles and/or energy from an unstable nucleus. The particles and/or energy that are emitted are referred to as *radiation.* The three types of radiation in nuclear chemistry are alpha, beta, and gamma.

Alpha radiation is the emission of helium nuclei. These particles contain two protons and two neutrons, causing them to have a charge of plus two (+2). Alpha particles are the largest of the radioactive emissions, and penetration from alpha particles can generally be stopped by a piece of paper.

Beta radiation is a product of the decomposition of a neutron or proton. It is actually composed of high-energy, high-speed electrons that began as neutrons or protons. These particles are either negatively charged (electrons) or positively charged (positrons). Because they have virtually no mass, beta particles can be stopped by a thin sheet of aluminum foil, Lucite, or plastic.

Gamma radiation is high-energy electromagnetic radiation, similar to x-rays but with more energy. It is very penetrating and can go through several feet of concrete or several inches of lead. Lead shielding is required to block gamma rays.

An isotope is written as an abbreviation with the symbol of the element preceded by a superscript number indicating the atomic mass. For example, Iodine-131 is correctly abbreviated as ^{131}I, and Iodine-125 would be written as ^{125}I. In nature, some isotopes are stable and some are unstable. Given enough time, unstable nuclei will change or "decay" into more stable forms. The amount of time it takes for half of the unstable isotope to decay is called the half-life. In nuclear chemistry, the unstable atom *decays* until it finds a stable nuclear configuration, usually by emitting radioactive particles. The amount of time used in a half-life ($T^{1/2}$) is different for every radioactive element. Some half-lives are very long, and some are as short as a few days. An example of radioactive half-life or decay is ^{131}I, which has a half-life of approximately 8 days, or every 8 days one-half of the radioactive particles will be emitted or decayed. This will happen over and over again until the ^{131}I reaches a stable nuclear configuration.

Biochemistry

Biochemistry is the study of chemical processes in living organisms. Much of biochemistry deals with the structures and functions of molecules such as carbohydrates, proteins, lipids, and nucleic acids.

Carbohydrates

Sugars and starches are carbohydrates. Their most important function is to store and provide energy for the body. The sugars **deoxyribose** and **ribose** are used in the formation of deoxyribonucleic acid (DNA) and ribonucleic acid (RNA), respectively. Carbohydrates are more abundant than any other known type of biomolecule.

The simplest type of carbohydrate is a **monosaccharide**. Monosaccharides contain carbon, hydrogen, and oxygen in a ratio of 1:2:1 (general formula $C_m(H_2O)n$, where m is at least three). Glucose ($C_6H_{12}O_6$) is one of the most important carbohydrates and is an example of a monosaccharide. Fructose ($C_6H_{12}O_6$), the sugar commonly associated with the sweet taste of fruits, is also a monosaccharide. Glucose and fructose are both a six-carbon sugar called a *hexose* (Fig. 6.5).

HESI Hint

The word "saccharide" comes from a Greek word meaning "sugar."

HESI Hint

Glucose and fructose have the same chemical formula ($C_6H_{12}O_6$) but different actual molecular configurations.

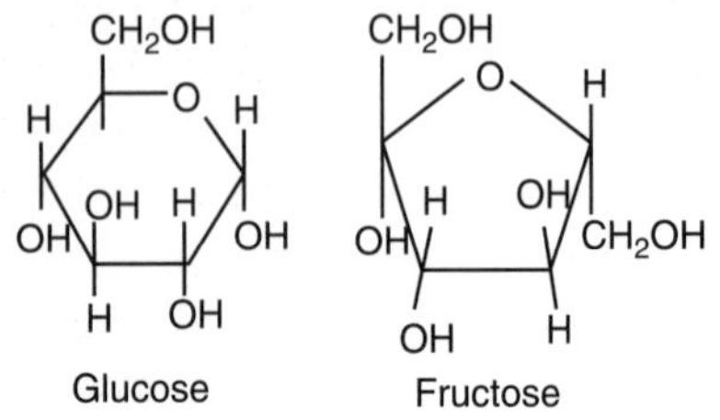

FIGURE 6.5 Molecular configuration for glucose and fructose.

Two monosaccharides can be joined together to make a **disaccharide**. The most well-known disaccharide is sucrose, which is ordinary sugar. Sucrose consists of a glucose molecule and a fructose molecule joined together. Another disaccharide is lactose, or milk sugar, consisting of a glucose molecule and a galactose molecule. Fig. 6.6 illustrates the molecular configuration of sucrose and lactose.

When three to six monosaccharides are joined together, it is called an **oligosaccharide** (oligo meaning "few"). More than six and up to thousands of monosaccharides joined together make a **polysaccharide**, which can be called a *starch*. Two of the most common polysaccharides are cellulose, made by plants, and glycogen, made by animals; both of these polysaccharides are chains of repeating glucose units.

Carbohydrates as Energy

Glycolysis Glucose is mainly metabolized by a chemical pathway in the body called glycolysis. The net result is the breakdown of one molecule of glucose into two molecules of pyruvate; this also produces a net two molecules of adenosine triphosphate (ATP). ATP is the substance cells use for energy. In aerobic cells with sufficient oxygen, like most human cells, the pyruvate is further metabolized by a process called *oxidative phosphorylation* (Krebs cycle) generating more molecules of ATP, water, and carbon dioxide. Using oxygen to completely oxidize glucose provides an organism with far more energy than any oxygen-deficient system.

When skeletal muscles are used in vigorous exercise, they will not have enough oxygen to meet their energy demands. They will need to use another type of glucose metabolism called anaerobic glycolysis. Anaerobic means in the absence of

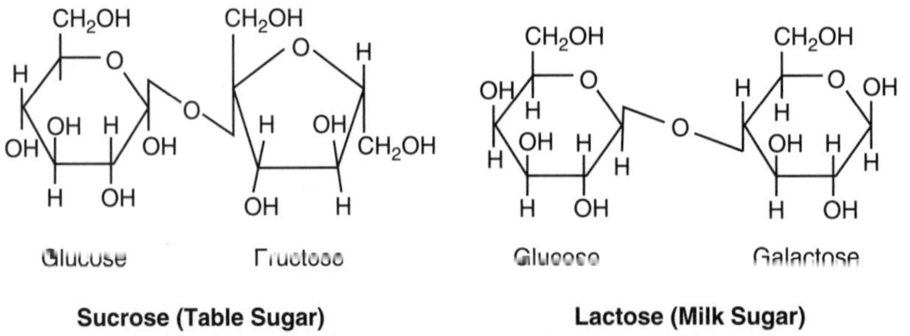

Sucrose (Table Sugar)   **Lactose (Milk Sugar)**

FIGURE 6.6 Molecular configuration for sucrose and lactose.

or without oxygen. This process converts glucose to lactate instead of pyruvate as in aerobic glycolysis. The production of lactate, an acid, in the muscles creates the "burning or cramping" sensation during intense exercise.

HESI Hint

An aerobic organism or cell requires oxygen to sustain life. An anaerobic organism or cell can function in low concentrations of oxygen, also called microaerobic, and some anaerobic organisms exist with no oxygen present.

Gluconeogenesis The liver can make glucose from other noncarbohydrate sources, such as proteins and parts of fats, using a process called gluconeogenesis. The glucose produced can then enter the energy-producing cycles mentioned previously and undergo glycolysis, or glucose can be stored as glycogen in animals or as cellulose in plants. Glucose can also be used to make other saccharides.

Proteins

Proteins are made up of amino acids. An amino acid is a molecule composed of a carbon atom bonded with four other groups: an amine group (NH_2), a carboxyl group (COOH), a hydrogen, and an R group (Fig. 6.7). The R group is different for each amino acid, giving each amino acid its own identity and characteristics. Amino acids are joined together to make proteins or parts of proteins. A union of two amino acids using a peptide bond is called a *dipeptide*; groups of fewer than 30 amino acids are called peptides or polypeptides. Larger groups are referred to as proteins. As an example, an important protein in blood called *albumin* contains 585 amino acid residues, and albumin is considered a fairly small protein. In humans, there are only 20 amino acids needed to make all the proteins necessary for life.

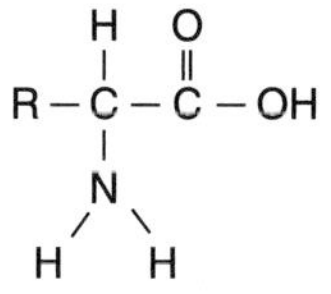

Lipids

Lipids are fats and encompass a large group of molecules, including oils, fats, and fatty acids. Fatty acids consist of a hydrocarbon chain with an acid group, the carboxyl group (COOH), at one end. A neutral fat (triglyceride) is three fatty acids generally joined to a glycerol or some other backbone structure (Fig. 6.8). Phospholipids are similar to neutral fats, but one of the three fatty acids is replaced by a phosphate group. Cholesterol is yet another form of fat composed of a four-ring structure and a side chain. Fats are used by the body to insulate body organs against shock, to maintain body temperature, to keep skin and hair healthy, and to promote healthy cell function. Phospholipids are essential components of cell membranes, and cholesterol is an obligatory precursor for many important biologic molecules such as steroid hormones. Fats also serve as energy stores for the body.

Lipids are found in many foods, such as oils, milk, and milk products such as butter and cheese. Natural lipids can be classified as unsaturated, polyunsaturated, and saturated. Saturated fats have no double bond between carbon atoms of the fatty acid chains (Fig. 6.9). Unsaturated fats have one or more double bonds between some of the carbon atoms of the fatty acid chains and are more desirable in our diet than saturated fats (Fig. 6.10).

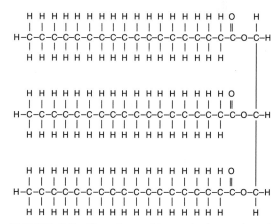

FIGURE 6.8 Three fatty acids attached to a glycerol.

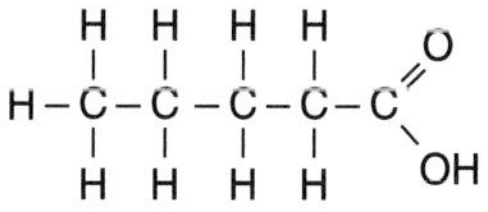

FIGURE 6.7 An amino acid general formula.

FIGURE 6.9 An example of a saturated fatty acid.

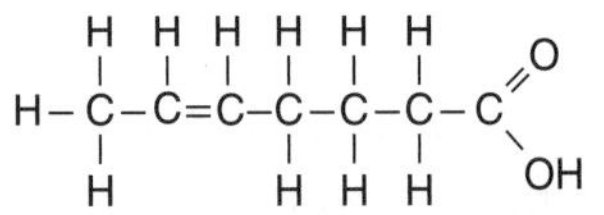

H–C=C=C–C–C–C–C=O / OH

FIGURE 6.10 An example of an unsaturated fatty acid. Note that there are two hydrogens missing, and there is a double bond, designated by two lines, between the two carbons in the center of the fatty acid.

Nucleic Acids

Nucleic acids are the biologic brain of life, telling the cell what it will do and how to do it. They include DNA and RNA. Both are nucleotide chains that convey genetic information. Nucleic acids are found in all living cells and viruses. Most nucleic acids are found in the nucleus, but some are found in the cytoplasm and mitochondria of individual cells. They are very large molecules that have two main parts.

The backbone of the molecule DNA is composed of deoxyribose, a five-carbon sugar that is also called a pentose, and a phosphate, which alternately chain together in a "sugar-phosphate-sugar-phosphate" chain, making two very long structures. The two chains, or strands, actually twist around each other like the strands of a rope, which is referred to as a "double helix."

The DNA bases adenine, cytosine, guanine, and thymine join the two chains from sugar to sugar much like the rungs of a ladder in a base pair relationship. The pair relationships are constant in that adenine and thymine are always bound together and cytosine and guanine are always bound together in DNA. Note that the two sugar-phosphate chains in DNA run in opposite directions: one up and one down. This is termed *anti-parallel*.

The structure of RNA differs from DNA's structure in that RNA is a single strand of ribose, a five-carbon carbohydrate, in a sugar-phosphate chain (Fig. 6.11). RNA does not use thymine to form one of its base pairs; it uses instead uracil to bind with adenine. Cytosine and guanine are the other base pair.

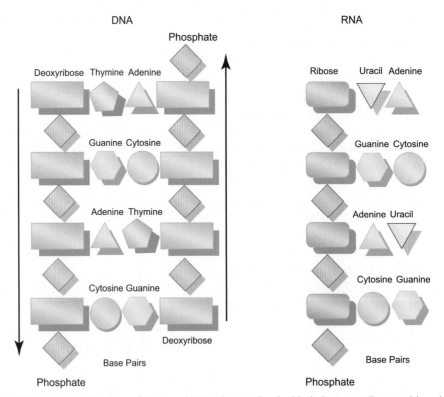

FIGURE 6.11 Structure of DNA and RNA. (Note: The double helix is not illustrated here.)

REVIEW QUESTIONS

1. An individual who weighs 70 kg weighs how many pounds?
   A. 154 lbs
   B. 140 lbs
   C. 35 lbs
   D. 32 lbs

2. How many protons does oxygen (O) have? (Refer to the periodic table.)
   A. 24
   B. 16
   C. 8
   D. 6

3. The atomic number of an atom is equal to the number of:
   A. Electrons
   B. Neutrons
   C. Protons
   D. Isotopes

4. Oxidation refers to the:
   A. Loss of electrons
   B. Sharing of electrons
   C. Gaining of electrons
   D. Unsharing of electrons

5. What are the weakest bonds between two molecules?
   A. Dispersion forces
   B. Dipole-dipole interactions
   C. Ionic bonds
   D. Hydrogen bonds

6. What effect does a catalyst have on a chemical reaction?
   A. Increases the temperature
   B. Decreases the activation energy
   C. Increases the activation energy
   D. Decreases the temperature

7. A temperature of 100°C represents the:
   A. Highest temperature achievable
   B. Normal body temperature
   C. Boiling point of water
   D. Melting point of ice

8. What term describes the decay of an unstable isotope?
   A. Half-life
   B. Decomposition
   C. Sublimation
   D. Reduction

9. Which of the following is an example of a double replacement reaction?
   A. $NaCl \rightarrow Na^+ + Cl^-$
   B. $Pb(NO_3)_2 + 2KI \rightarrow 2KNO_3 + PbI_2$
   C. $2Na + 2HCl \rightarrow 2NaCl + H_2$
   D. $2C_2H_6 + 7O_2 \rightarrow 4CO_2 + 6H_2O$

10. What is the correct coefficient for the products of the following reaction when the equation is balanced? $C_6H_{12}O_6 + 6O_2 \rightarrow \_\_CO_2 + \_\_H_2O$
    A. 2
    B. 4
    C. 6
    D. 8

11. Which of the following increases the rate of a chemical reaction?
    A. Increasing the activation energy
    B. Decreasing the surface area
    C. Decreasing the concentration
    D. Increasing the temperature

12. What type of reaction involves the breaking of a compound into separate components?
    A. Replacement
    B. Combustion
    C. Synthesis
    D. Decomposition

13. Which molecule can act as both an acid and a base?
    A. HCl
    B. H_2O
    C. NaCl
    D. NaOH

14. Which chemical pathway produces the greatest amount of ATP?
    A. Aerobic glycolysis
    B. Anaerobic glycolysis
    C. Gluconeogenesis
    D. Oxidative phosphorylation

15. What exponent is equal to 10,000?
    A. 10^6
    B. 10^5
    C. 10^4
    D. 10^3

16. What macromolecules are responsible for passing on genetic information?
  A. Proteins
  B. Nucleic acids
  C. Carbohydrates
  D. Lipids

17. Which term refers to a chain of 100 or more amino acids joined together?
  A. Protein
  B. Dipeptide
  C. Peptide
  D. Polypeptide

ANSWERS TO REVIEW QUESTIONS

1. A
2. C
3. C
4. A
5. A
6. B
7. C
8. A
9. B

10. C
11. D
12. D
13. B
14. D
15. C
16. B
17. A

ANATOMY AND PHYSIOLOGY

7

From cells and tissues to organs and systems, the human body is one of the most complex organisms on earth. Members of health professions who take care of patients need to know how the human body works as a whole, and what role specific parts of the body play in an individual's health and well-being. This information is the basis for understanding conditions, diseases, and dysfunctions, and for determining which treatments are most appropriate for the patient.

A 1-year course in anatomy and physiology should be undertaken before the student prepares for the anatomy and physiology examination. Additionally, taking time to study anatomy and physiology at every opportunity is excellent preparation. This guide discusses each of the major body systems and emphasizes the most important information to know.

CHAPTER OUTLINE

KEY TERMS

Acetylcholine
Action Potential
Anatomical Position
Anterior (Ventral)
Appendicular Skeleton
Autonomic Nervous System
Axial Skeleton
Body Planes
Brainstem
Caudal
Cells
Cerebellum
Cerebrum
Contralateral
Cranial
Deep
Dermis
Diencephalon
Distal
Endocardium

Endosteum
Epidermis
Erythrocytes
External Respiration
Filtration
Hemopoiesis
Histology
Inferior
Internal Respiration
Ipsilateral
Lateral
Leukocytes
Medial
Myocardium
Myofibrils
Nephrons
Neuroglia
Neurons
Osteoblasts
Osteoclasts

Osteocytes
Osteogenic Cells
Pericardium
Periosteum
Posterior (Dorsal)
Proximal
Reabsorption
Remodeling
Saltatory Conduction
Sarcolemma
Sarcomeres
Sarcoplasmic Reticulum
Secretion
Sliding Filament Model
Superficial
Superior
Thrombocytes
Troponin-Tropomyosin Complex

General Terminology

Standard terminology is used across all health professions to facilitate common understanding. This terminology includes directions for locating structures on and within the body, as well as for subdivisions and regions of the body.

Anatomical position provides a baseline reference point for areas of the body. In this position, the body is erect, the feet are slightly apart, the head is held upright, the arms are at the sides, and the palms of the hands are facing forward.

Body planes are imaginary lines that divide the body at particular angles. A sagittal plane is a vertical plane that divides the body or body part into right and left sides. The midsagittal plane divides the body into equal right and left halves. A frontal (coronal) plane is a vertical plane that divides the body or body part into front (anterior) and back (posterior) sections. A transverse plane is a horizontal plane that divides the body or body part into upper (superior) and lower (inferior)

sections. An oblique plane is any plane that intersects the body at an angle other than vertical or horizontal.

Directional terms to review include **superior** (above), **inferior** (below), **anterior/ventral** (toward the front), **posterior/dorsal** (toward the back), **medial** (toward the midline), and **lateral** (away from the midline). **Cranial** means toward the head, and **caudal** means toward the tail (away from the head). **Ipsilateral** refers to something located or occurring on the same side of the body, and **contralateral** refers to something on the opposite side of the body. **Proximal** and **distal** are terms of direction that are often used in reference to the extremities. Proximal means closer to the point of attachment of the extremity to the trunk, and distal refers to farther away from the point of attachment of the extremity to the trunk. Figure 7.1 depicts planes and directional terms. Additionally, **superficial** means closer to or at the surface of the body, and **deep** means further into the body.

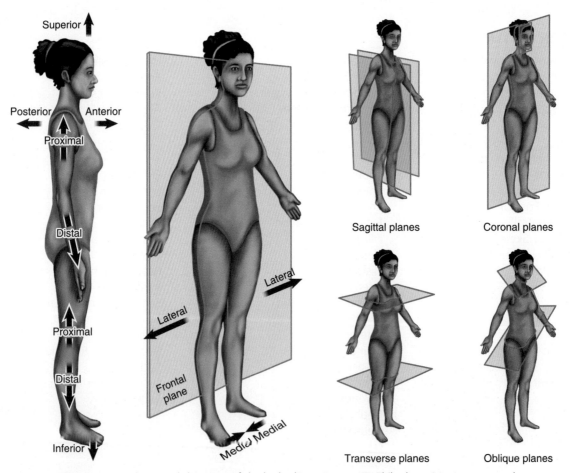

FIGURE 7.1 Planes and directions of the body. (From Patton KT, Thibodeau GA: *Anatomy and physiology*, ed 9, St Louis, 2016, Mosby.)

The major body cavities are the dorsal cavity, which includes the cranial and spinal cavities, and the ventral cavity, which includes the thoracic and abdominopelvic cavities. The thoracic cavity includes two pleural cavities, which contain the lungs, and the pericardial cavity, which contains the heart. The abdominopelvic cavity is further divided into the abdominal cavity and the pelvic cavity. The abdominal cavity contains the digestive organs, and the pelvic cavity contains the reproductive organs, the urinary bladder, and the lower gastrointestinal tract.

The joints of the body are capable of many types of movement. Health professionals use specific terms to describe the various body movements (Table 7.1).

Histology

Histology is the study of tissues. A tissue is a group of cells that act together to perform specific functions. The four types of tissues are epithelial, connective, muscle, and nervous (Fig. 7.2). Epithelial tissue covers, lines, and protects the body and its internal organs. Glandular epithelium secretes substances such as mucus, enzymes, and hormones. Connective tissue is the most abundant tissue in the body. It forms the framework of the body, providing support and structure for the organs. Types include fibrous (areolar, adipose, reticular, dense), bone, cartilage, and blood.

Nervous tissue is composed of **neurons**, which initiate and conduct nerve impulses, and connective tissue cells called **neuroglia**, which support the neurons. Muscle tissue has the ability to contract or shorten, as well as to lengthen. The three types of muscle tissue are described later in the chapter.

Integumentary System

The integumentary system consists of the skin and its structures and organs such as hair, nails, and sensory receptors. The skin is the largest organ of the body. Its structure is illustrated in Figure 7.3.

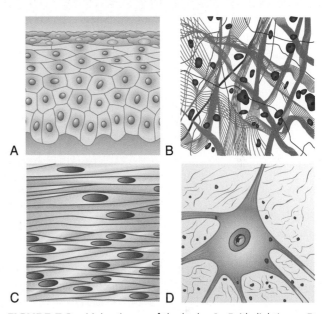

FIGURE 7.2 Major tissues of the body. **A,** Epithelial tissue; **B,** connective tissue; **C,** muscle tissue; **D,** nervous tissue. (From Patton KT, Thibodeau GA: *Anatomy and physiology,* ed 9, St Louis, 2016, Mosby.)

Table 7.1 Terms Used to Describe Types of Body Movements	
Term	**Movement**
Flexion	Bending of a joint
Extension	Straightening of a joint
Abduction	Moving away from the midline
Adduction	Moving toward the midline
Medial (internal) rotation	Rotating toward the midline
Lateral (external) rotation	Rotating away from the midline
Pronation	Rotating the forearm so the palm faces down
Supination	Rotating the forearm so the palm faces up
Dorsiflexion	Decreasing the angle between the top of the foot and the front of the leg
Plantar flexion	Decreasing the angle between the bottom of the foot and the back of the leg
Inversion	Turning the sole of the foot inward toward the midline
Eversion	Turning the sole of the foot outward away from the midline

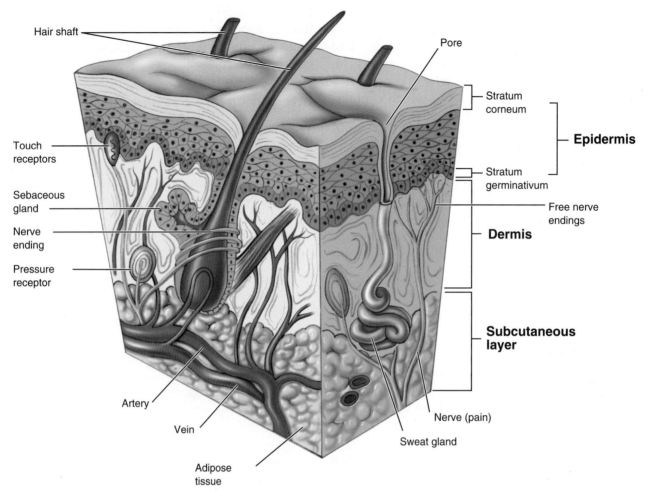

FIGURE 7.3 Diagram of skin structure. (From Herlihy B: *The human body in health and illness,* ed 5, St Louis, 2014, Saunders.)

The outer layer of skin is the **epidermis**, which is a protective layer made of dead, keratinized epithelial cells. The underlying layer of connective tissue is the **dermis.** The dermis rests on a subcutaneous layer known as the hypodermis, or superficial fascia, which connects the skin to underlying muscles and bones.

The layers of the epidermis from superficial to deep are the stratum corneum, stratum lucidum, stratum granulosum, stratum spinosum, and stratum germinativum (stratum basale), which continually undergoes mitosis. Epidermal cells contain *keratin*, which waterproofs the skin, and melanocytes, which produce a pigment called *melanin* that darkens the skin and protects against radiation from the sun.

The dermis is composed of fibrous connective tissue and contains blood vessels, sensory nerve endings, hair follicles, and glands. There are two types of sweat glands. Eccrine sweat glands are the most widely distributed. Eccrine glands help cool the body by releasing a watery secretion that evaporates from the surface of the skin. Apocrine sweat glands are mainly found in the axilla and inguinal regions. Sweat produced by apocrine glands is thicker because it contains bits of cytoplasm from the secreting cells. This cell debris attracts bacteria, and the presence of the bacteria on the skin results in body odor.

Sebaceous glands release an oily secretion called *sebum*, which is released through the hair follicles in order to lubricate and moisturize the skin. These glands are susceptible to becoming clogged and attracting bacteria, particularly during adolescence, resulting in acne. The appendages of the skin include hair and nails. Both are composed of plates of keratin. Certain diseases cause changes in the hair, nails, and skin; therefore, careful observation of the integumentary system is necessary when diagnosing clinical conditions. For example, melanoma is a cancer associated with the skin. Blue-tinged nails can indicate lack of adequate blood oxygenation. Thin, brittle hair may indicate malnutrition.

HESI Hint

As the epidermal cells move from the deepest layers to the superficial layers, they move away from their blood and nutrient supply; subsequently, they dehydrate and die. To illustrate this, visualize a large transparent container filled with inflated balloons covered with sticky glue. This illustrates the stratum basale. As the balloons deflate, the sides that are stuck together pull the balloons into a spiny shape, much like the stratum spinosum. As the balloons continue to deflate, they become flattened, like the stratum corneum.

Skeletal System

The body framework consists of bone, cartilage, ligaments, and joints. Functions of the skeletal system include support, movement, blood cell formation (**hemopoiesis**), protection of internal organs, and storage of minerals (especially calcium and phosphorus).

The two types of bone tissue are compact (dense) and spongy (cancellous). Compact bone forms the hard outer layer of all bones. The inner spongy layer contains plates of bone called trabeculae. Spaces between the trabeculae are filled with red marrow, which produces red blood cells, white blood cells, and platelets.

Compact bone is covered by the periosteal membrane, or **periosteum**. The periosteum consists of an external fibrous layer containing blood vessels and nerves, and an inner layer that consists of bone-forming cells. The **endosteum** is a thin, vascular connective tissue layer that lines the cavities of bones. The periosteum and endosteum contain cells responsible for building and remodeling bones.

Individual bones are classified by shape. The classifications include long bones, short bones, flat bones, irregular bones, and sesamoid bones. A typical long bone has an *epiphysis* at each end, which is composed mainly of spongy bone covered by compact bone. The shaft of a long bone is called the *diaphysis*. It is composed mainly of compact bone surrounding a hollow center called the *medullary cavity*. The medullary cavity is filled with yellow marrow, which is mostly fat. The widened area between the epiphysis and

diaphysis is called the *metaphysis*. During childhood, the metaphysis contains the *epiphyseal plate* (growth plate). This is where longitudinal bone growth takes place. During adolescence, the epiphyseal plate begins to close, at which point it becomes the *epiphyseal line*. The features of a typical long bone are demonstrated in Figure 7.4.

Bone Cells

Osteoblasts are cells that form new bone. Osteoblasts are derived from **osteogenic cells**. Osteogenic cells are located in the periosteum and endosteum, and are the only bone cells capable of dividing. When bone formation is complete, some

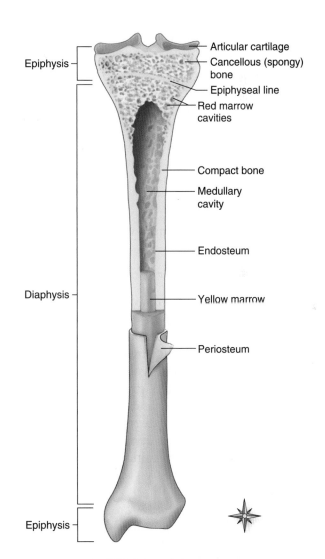

FIGURE 7.4 Anatomy of a long bone. (From Patton KT, Thibodeau GA: *The human body in health & disease*, ed 7, St. Louis, 2018, Elsevier.)

of the osteoblasts become trapped in the bone matrix. Once imbedded in the matrix, osteoblasts become **osteocytes**, or mature bone cells. **Osteoclasts** are derived from white blood cells called monocytes and are responsible for breaking down and resorbing old bone tissue. **Remodeling** is the continuous process of old bone being broken down by osteoclasts and replaced with stronger bone by osteoblasts.

Bone Repair

When a bone is fractured, the body sends out signals that trigger a four-stage healing process. The first stage is *hematoma formation*, which occurs when ruptured vessels bleed in and around the fracture site. Blood clots form to stop further leakage of blood from damaged vessels. Clotting cuts off the blood supply to surrounding bone cells and causes these cells to die. The second stage is *bone generation*. In this stage, phagocytic white blood cells arrive at the fracture site to remove the blood clots and dead cells. Once the debris is removed and blood flow is restored, osteoblasts and fibroblasts work together to form a soft callus of fibrocartilage between the two broken ends. The third stage is *bony callus formation*, during which the soft callus is replaced by spongy bone. Finally, *bone remodeling* occurs as osteoclasts resorb the old bone and osteoblasts form new bone.

Joints: Structure and Function

The area where two bones meet is a joint. All joints belong to one of three *functional* categories: synarthrotic (immovable), amphiarthrotic (slightly movable), and diarthrotic (freely moveable). The degree of movement is inversely related to the stability of the joint: the greater the range of movement, the less stable (and prone to injury) the joint is. Joints are also categorized according to structure. The three *structural* classifications of joints are fibrous, cartilaginous, and synovial. Table 7.2 summarizes the two ways in which joints are classified.

Most joints in the body are synovial joints (Fig. 7.5). All synovial joints are diarthroses (freely movable), but they differ in the type and degree of movement. Unlike fibrous and cartilaginous joints, synovial joints are surrounded by an *articular capsule* made up of two layers: an outer fibrous

Table 7.2 Functional and Structural Classifications of Joints

Functional Classifications (Degree of Movement)	Structural Classifications (Type of Tissue)
• Synarthrotic (immovable) • Amphiarthrotic (slightly movable) • Diarthrotic (freely movable)	• Fibrous • Cartilaginous • Synovial

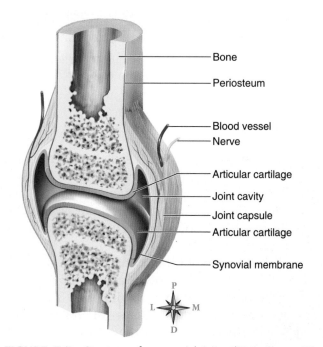

FIGURE 7.5 Structure of a synovial joint. (From Patton KT, Thibodeau GA: *The human body in health & disease*, ed 7, St. Louis, 2018, Elsevier.)

layer that provides stability, and an inner synovial layer that produces *synovial fluid* to reduce friction during movement. The articulating surfaces of the bones are covered by a thin layer of *articular cartilage* that absorbs shock and allows for smooth movement. Articular cartilage has no blood supply, but it receives nourishment from the synovial fluid. The six types of synovial joints are hinge, pivot, gliding, ball and socket, condylar, and saddle (Fig. 7.6).

The Skeleton

The **axial skeleton** (Fig. 7.7) consists of the skull, vertebral column, 12 pairs of ribs, and sternum When including the six paired bones (ossicles) of the ear, the skull comprises 28 bones—14 facial

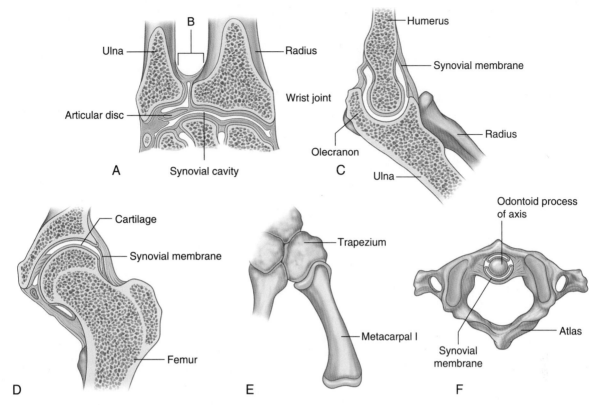

FIGURE 7.6 Types of synovial joints. **A,** Condylar (wrist). **B,** Gliding (radio-ulnar). **C,** Hinge (elbow). **D,** Ball and socket (hip). **E,** Saddle (carpometacarpal of thumb). **F,** Pivot (atlanto-axial). (From Drake RL, Vogl W, Mitchell AWM: *Gray's anatomy for students,* ed 5, Elsevier, 2024.)

bones and 14 cranial vault bones. The facial bones include two nasal bones, two maxillary bones, two zygomatic bones, one mandible (the only movable bone of the skull), two palatine bones, one vomer, two lacrimal bones, and two inferior nasal conchae. The bones of the cranium are single occipital, frontal, ethmoid, and sphenoid bones, and the paired parietal and temporal bones. The ossicles of the ear (malleus, incus, and stapes) are part of the skull.

The vertebral column is divided into five subsections, as depicted in Figure 7.8. There are seven cervical vertebrae, twelve thoracic vertebrae, five lumbar vertebrae, five sacral vertebrae (which fuse to form the sacrum), and the fused coccygeal vertebrae (known as the tailbone).

The **appendicular skeleton** (see Fig. 7.7) includes the shoulder girdles, hip girdles, and the extremities. The upper portion consists of the pectoral or shoulder girdles (formed by the clavicles and scapulae), and the upper extremities. The bones of the arm are the humerus, radius and ulna, carpals (wrist bones), metacarpals (bones of the hand), and phalanges (bones of the fingers). The lower appendicular skeleton is made up of the pelvic girdle, which is formed by the right and left os coxae (hip bones), and the lower extremities. Both os coxae consist of a fused ilium, ischium, and pubis. Bones of the lower extremity include the femur (thigh bone), tibia and fibula, tarsals (ankle bones), metatarsals (bones of the foot), and phalanges (bones of the toes).

Muscular System

The muscular system (Fig. 7.9) consists of three types of muscle tissue: skeletal, cardiac, and smooth. Skeletal muscles are called voluntary muscles because they are mostly under conscious control. Skeletal muscle cells are multinucleated, cylindrical, and have a striated appearance. Cardiac muscle is under involuntary control. Cardiac muscle cells are mononucleated, cylindrical, and striated. The cells of cardiac muscle are connected by *intercalated discs,* which help propagate nerve

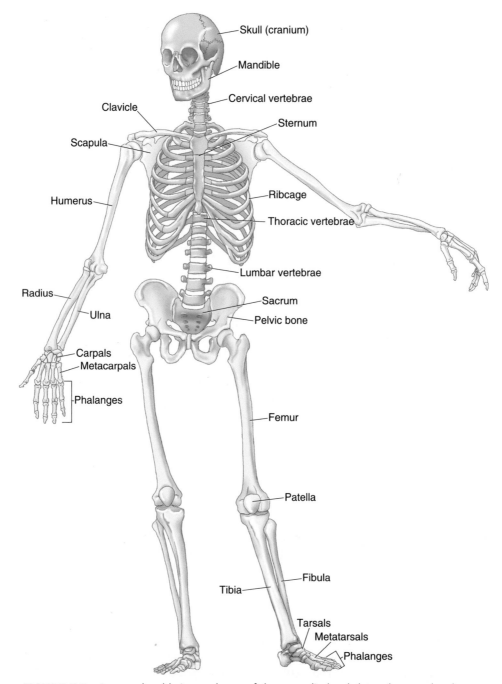

Skull (cranium)

Mandible

Cervical vertebrae

Sternum

Clavicle

Scapula

Ribcage

Humerus

Thoracic vertebrae

Lumbar vertebrae

Radius

Sacrum

Ulna

Pelvic bone

Carpals
Metacarpals

Phalanges

Femur

Patella

Fibula

Tibia

Tarsals
Metatarsals
Phalanges

FIGURE 7.7 Bones colored beige are bones of the appendicular skeleton; bones colored green are bones of the axial skeleton. (From Muscolino JE: *Kinesiology: the skeletal system and muscle function*, ed 2, St Louis, 2011, Mosby.)

impulses throughout the myocardium. Smooth muscles are involuntary muscles that line the walls of blood vessels and hollow organs. Smooth muscle cells are mononucleated, spindle-shaped, and nonstriated. Figure 7.10 shows the three types of muscle tissue.

Muscles produce movement by contracting in response to nervous stimulation. When the nervous system generates a signal, or **action potential**, the signal travels through the axon of a motor neuron until it reaches the axon terminal, or nerve ending. The motor neuron then releases a neurotransmitter called **acetylcholine**, which diffuses across the gap between the nerve cell and the muscle cell and causes depolarization of the muscle cell membrane, or **sarcolemma**. Depolarization of the sarcolemma triggers the release of stored calcium ions from the **sarcoplasmic reticulum**.

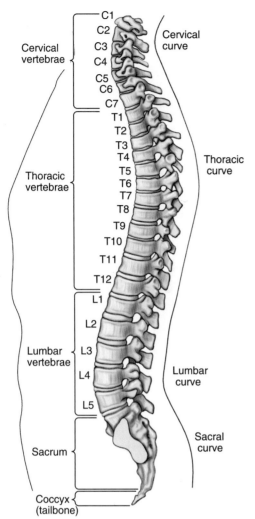

Cervical vertebrae

C1
C2
C3
C4
C5
C6
C7

Cervical curve

Thoracic vertebrae

T1
T2
T3
T4
T5
T6
T7
T8
T9
T10
T11
T12

Thoracic curve

Lumbar vertebrae

L1
L2
L3
L4
L5

Lumbar curve

Sacrum

Sacral curve

Coccyx (tailbone)

FIGURE 7.8 Vertebral column. (From Herlihy B: *The human body in health and illness*, ed 5, St Louis, 2014, Saunders.)

Muscle Contraction

Each muscle cell, or muscle fiber, consists of **myofibrils** divided into contractile units called **sarcomeres**. Sarcomeres contain the myofilaments *actin*, a thin protein, and *myosin*, a thick protein. (The arrangement of actin and myosin filaments gives skeletal muscle its striated appearance.) Muscle contraction is produced by the binding of these two filaments. The binding sites on actin are regulated by an arrangement of proteins called the **troponin-tropomyosin complex**. Troponin covers the binding sites on the actin filament, while troponin holds the tropomyosin in place. When calcium is released from the sarcoplasmic reticulum in striated muscle cells, the calcium ions bind to troponin and move tropomyosin out of the way so that the myosin head can attach to the binding sites on actin. Muscle contraction occurs as myosin moves along the binding sites on the actin filament, pulling it toward the center and shortening the sarcomere. This process is called the **sliding filament model**.

Nervous System

The nervous system consists of the brain, spinal cord, and nerves (Fig. 7.11). The two main divisions of the nervous system are the central nervous system (CNS), which is made up of the spinal cord and brain, and the peripheral nervous system (PNS), which is made up of the cranial nerves and peripheral nerves. The PNS consists of sensory (afferent) neurons and motor (efferent) neurons. Afferent neurons transmit nerve impulses toward the CNS, and efferent neurons transmit nerve impulses away from the CNS toward effector organs (e.g., muscles, glands, and digestive organs).

The PNS is subdivided into the somatic system and the autonomic system. The somatic nervous system allows voluntary muscle control and processes sensory information from the skin, muscles, bones, and joints. The **autonomic nervous system** controls functions such as digestion, heart rate, blood pressure, and urination. The two divisions of the autonomic nervous system are the *parasympathetic division* ("rest and digest") and the *sympathetic division* ("fight or flight"). Figure 7.12 shows the divisions of the nervous system.

The Brain

The brain consists of four major parts. The **cerebrum** is the largest part of the brain and is associated with sensory interpretation, movement, thinking, and personality. The **cerebellum** is responsible for muscular coordination. The **diencephalon** contains the thalamus, which routes incoming sensory information to the appropriate part of the cerebrum, and the hypothalamus, which monitors many of the conditions of the body, controls the autonomic nervous system, and interacts with the endocrine system. The **brainstem** connects the brain with the spinal cord and controls many vital functions such as respiration and heart rate. The superior section of the brainstem is called the midbrain, the middle section is the pons, and the inferior portion is called the medulla oblongata. Deep inside the brain are four

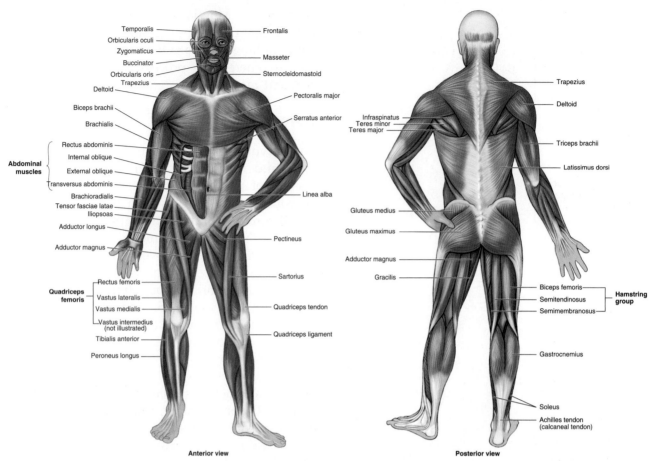

FIGURE 7.9   General overview of the body's musculature (anterior and posterior view). (From Herlihy B: *The human body in health and illness,* ed 5, St Louis, 2014, Saunders.)

ventricles that produce cerebrospinal fluid, which provides a cushion for the brain and spinal cord.

Spinal Cord

The spinal cord is housed within the vertebral columns and extends from the brainstem to the level of the first or second lumbar vertebra (L1 or L2). The tapered inferior end of the spinal cord is called the *conus medullaris.* The conus medullaris is attached to the coccyx by a thin fibrous filament called the filum terminale, which acts as an anchor for the distal end of the spinal cord. Thirty-one pairs of spinal nerves exit the spinal cord. A bundle of spinal nerves extends below the conus medullaris to form the *cauda equina.* The spinal cord is surrounded by three protective layers called meninges. The outer layer is called the dura mater, the middle layer is the arachnoid matter, and the inner layer is the pia mater. The cerebrospinal fluid that surrounds the spinal cord

flows through the *subarachnoid space,* which is the space between the arachnoid mater and the pia mater.

Nerve Conduction

All actions of the nervous system depend on the transmission of nerve impulses along the neurons. The main parts of a neuron are the cell body (soma), axon, and dendrites. Dendrites transmit the impulse toward the cell body, and axons transmit the impulse away from the cell body. PNS axons are covered by an insulating layer called the *myelin sheath,* which greatly increases the speed of the action potential. Unmyelinated gaps along the myelin sheath called the *nodes of Ranvier* reproduce the action potential along the axon. This arrangement of myelinated and un-myelinated segments along the axon allows the action potential to "jump" quickly from node to node by a process called **saltatory conduction.**

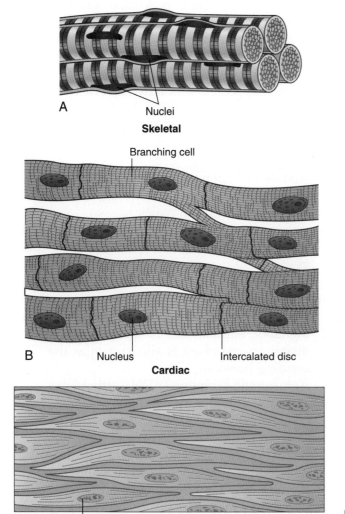

Skeletal

Cardiac

Smooth

FIGURE 7.10 Types of muscle tissue. **A,** Skeletal muscle fibers. **B,** Cardiac muscle fibers. **C,** Smooth muscle fibers. (From Waugh A, Grant A. *Ross & Wilson anatomy and physiology in health and illness*, ed 14, 2023, St. Louis, Elsevier.)

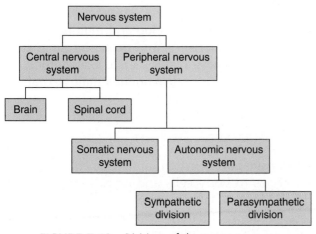

FIGURE 7.12 Divisions of the nervous system.

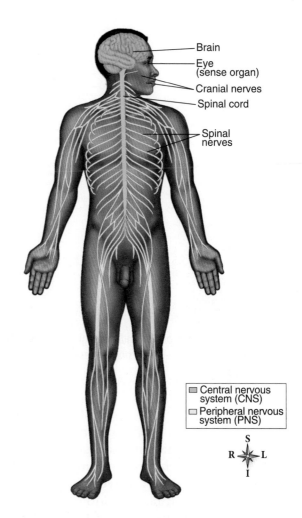

FIGURE 7.11 Major anatomical features of the nervous system include the brain, the spinal cord, and the individual nerves. The central nervous system consists of the brain and spinal cord. The peripheral nervous system includes all of the nerves and their branches. (From Patton KT, Thibodeau GA: *Anatomy and physiology*, ed 9, St Louis, 2016, Mosby.)

Endocrine System

The nervous and endocrine systems coordinate and control the body, but the endocrine system has more long-lasting and widespread effects. It also plays important roles in growth and sexual maturation. These two systems meet at the hypothalamus and pituitary gland. The hypothalamus governs the pituitary and is in turn controlled by the feedback of hormones in the blood as well as other conditions in the body. The endocrine glands, although widely distributed, are grouped together as a system because the main function of each gland is the production of hormones. Figure 7.13 shows the locations of the endocrine

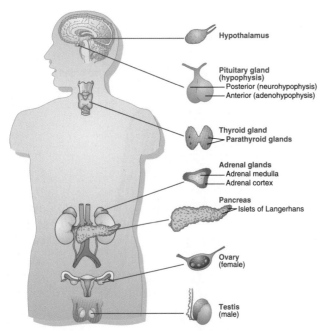

FIGURE 7.13 Locations of the endocrine glands. (From Kee: *Pharmacology: a patient-centered nursing process approach*, ed 8, St Louis, 2015, Saunders.)

glands. Other organs, such as the stomach, small intestine, and kidneys, produce hormones as well.

Hormones are chemical messengers that control the growth, differentiation, and metabolism of specific target cells. There are two major groups of hormones, steroid and nonsteroid hormones. Steroid hormones enter the target cells and have a direct effect on the DNA of the nucleus. Nonsteroid hormones remain at the cell surface and act through a second messenger, usually a substance called *adenosine monophosphate*, AMP. Most hormones affect cell activity by altering the rate of protein synthesis.

HESI Hint

Multiple hormones are released during stress from the adrenal cortex, the hypothalamus, and the anterior and posterior pituitary gland. Cortisol, released from the adrenal cortex, is sometimes called the "stress hormone" because it reduces inflammation, raises the blood sugar level, and inhibits the release of histamine during long-term stress.

The pituitary gland is attached to the hypothalamus by a stalk called the *infundibulum*. The pituitary gland has two major portions: the anterior lobe (adenohypophysis) and the posterior lobe (neurohypophysis). Hormones of the adenohypophysis are called *tropic hormones* because they act mainly on other endocrine glands. They include:

- Somatotropin hormone (STH) or growth hormone (GH)—stimulates growth in all organs.
- Adrenocorticotropic hormone (ACTH)—stimulates secretion of adrenal cortex hormones.
- Thyroid-stimulating hormone (TSH)—stimulates secretion of thyroid hormones.
- Follicle-stimulating hormone (FSH)—stimulates secretion of ovarian follicles and secretion of estrogens in females; stimulates sperm production in males.
- Luteinizing hormone (LH)—triggers ovulation in females; stimulates secretion of testosterone in males.

Hormones released from the posterior lobe of the pituitary include:

- Oxytocin—stimulates uterine contractions during labor; stimulates milk ejection from the mammary glands; it is also known as the bonding hormone.
- Antidiuretic hormone (ADH)—stimulates retention of water by the kidneys.

Other important endocrine glands include:

- Thyroid gland—secretes thyroid hormones which regulate metabolism, and calcitonin which decreases blood calcium levels.
- Parathyroid glands—secrete parathyroid hormone which increases blood calcium levels.
- Adrenal glands—cortex secretes cortisol (discussed in the HESI Hint); medulla secretes adrenaline which intensifies the sympathetic response.
- Pancreas—secretes insulin which decreases blood glucose levels, and glucagon which increases blood glucose levels.
- Gonads—ovaries secrete estrogens and progesterone. Estrogens develop and maintain female sexual characteristics, and progesterone maintains pregnancy. Testes secrete testosterone, which develops and maintains male sexual characteristics.

Cardiovascular System

Blood transports oxygen, nutrients, enzymes, and hormones to body cells and carries away carbon dioxide and metabolic wastes. Whole blood consists of approximately 55% plasma (the liquid portion). The remaining 45% is made up of formed elements, which include **erythrocytes** (red blood cells), **leukocytes** (white blood cells), and cell fragments called **thrombocytes** (platelets). All of the formed elements are produced from stem cells in red bone marrow.

Erythrocytes contain hemoglobin, which is made of protein and iron, and its function is to transport oxygen. When red blood cells die, the heme group of hemoglobin is broken down into a yellowish pigment called bilirubin, which is then converted into bile in the liver and excreted from the body.

Leukocytes are distinguished on the basis of size, appearance of the nucleus, staining properties, and the presence or absence of visible cytoplasmic granules. Granular leukocytes are neutrophils, basophils, and eosinophils. They are involved in phagocytosis, defense against parasites, and inflammation. Agranular leukocytes are lymphocytes and monocytes. They are involved in antibody production, cellular immune responses, and phagocytosis. Platelets are active in the process of blood clotting.

The Heart

The heart is surrounded by a fluid-filled sac called the **pericardium**. The pericardium consists of an outer (parietal) layer and an inner (visceral) layer. The inner layer of pericardium, also called the epicardium, is a serous membrane that forms the outermost layer of the heart wall. The middle layer of the heart is the **myocardium**, which is composed of cardiac muscle tissue. The myocardium receives its blood supply from the coronary arteries, which drain directly into the right atrium through the coronary sinus. The innermost layer of the heart is the **endocardium**, which forms the thin inner lining of the heart chambers and covers the heart valves.

Blood Circulation Through the Heart

The heart acts as a double pump that sends blood to the lungs for oxygenation through the pulmonary circuit, and to the remainder of the body through the systemic circuit. The superior and inferior vena cava deliver deoxygenated blood from the body to the right atrium, which sends it to the right ventricle. The right ventricle pumps this blood into the pulmonary arteries, which travel to the lungs. The blood becomes oxygenated in the lungs and travels through the pulmonary veins into the left atrium. The oxygenated blood then enters the left ventricle, which pumps it into the aorta to be transported throughout the body.

Heart Valves

When blood exits one of the chambers of the heart, it passes through one of four valves. Each heart valve prevents blood from flowing backward into the chamber. The tricuspid valve is between the right atrium and right ventricle; the bicuspid or mitral valve is between the left atrium and left ventricle. The pulmonary semilunar valve is located between the right ventricle and pulmonary trunk (which splits into the right and left main pulmonary arteries). The aortic semilunar valve is located between the left ventricle and the aorta.

Heart Conduction System

The heart has an intrinsic beat initiated by the sinoatrial node and transmitted along the conduction system through the myocardium. This wave of electrical activity is measured on an electrocardiogram (ECG). The cardiac cycle is the period from the end of one ventricular contraction to the end of the next ventricular contraction. The contraction phase of the cycles is called systole; the relaxation phase is called diastole.

HESI Hint

Deflections of the ECG do not represent the actual systole and diastole of the heart chambers. Instead, they represent the electrical activity that precedes the contraction-relaxation events of the myocardium. An analogy for this is the situation at a track meet when the starter's gun is fired before the runners start to run. The sound initiates the action. In the heart, the action potential is similar to firing the gun. The contraction starts just after the action potential passes over the muscle cells.

Blood Vessels

The cardiovascular system includes arteries that carry oxygenated blood away from the heart, veins that carry deoxygenated blood toward the heart, and capillaries. Capillaries, the smallest of vessels, are the sites of exchange of water, nutrients, and waste products between the blood and surrounding tissues. The systemic arteries begin with the aorta, which sends branches to all parts of the body. As arteries get farther away from the heart, they become thinner and thinner. The smallest arteries are called arterioles. Small veins called venules drain blood from the capillaries and send it to the veins. The veins parallel the arteries and most have the same names. The superior and inferior venae cava are the large veins that empty into the right atrium of the heart.

The walls of the arteries are thick and elastic, and they carry blood under high pressure. Vasoconstriction and vasodilation result from contraction and relaxation of smooth muscle in the arterial walls. These changes influence blood pressure and blood distribution to the tissues. The walls of the veins are thinner and less elastic than those of the arteries, and they carry blood under

lower pressure. Figure 7.14 provides an overall view of the cardiovascular system.

Respiratory System

The upper respiratory system consists of the nasal passages, pharynx, and larynx. The pharynx, which is also part of the digestive tract, provides passage for air, food, and drink. The larynx acts as a valve that prevents food and liquid from passing from the pharynx into the lower respiratory tract. The lower respiratory system includes the lungs and bronchial tree. The bronchial tree begins at the trachea, which extends from the bottom of the larynx and terminates at the *carina*. At the carina, the trachea branches into the right and left main bronchi. Each bronchus branches off into smaller airways called bronchioles, which lead

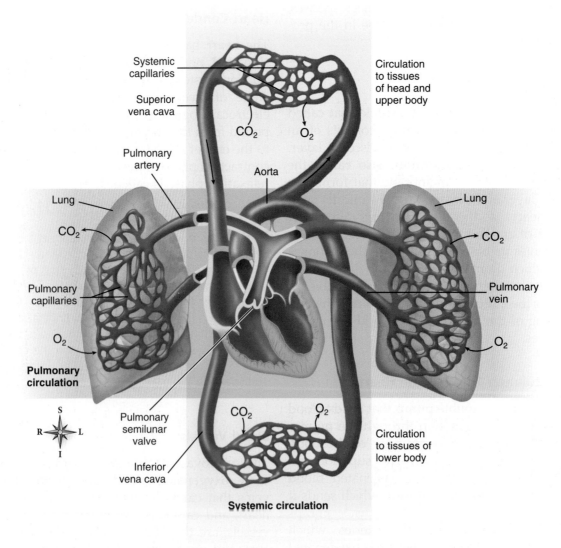

FIGURE 7.14 Principal arteries of the body. (From Patton KT, Thibodeau GA: *Structure & function of the body*, ed 15, St Louis, 2016, Elsevier.)

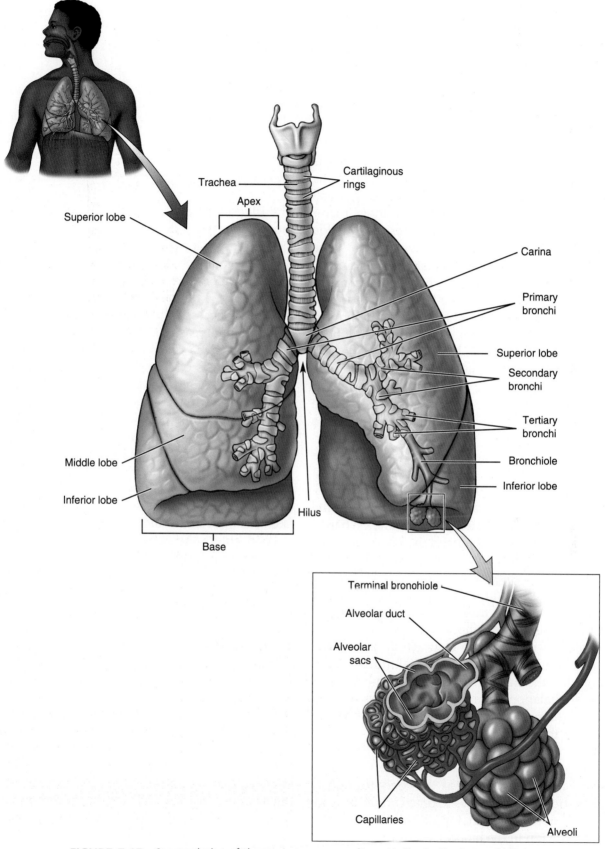

FIGURE 7.15 Structural plan of the respiratory system. (From Herlihy B: *The human body in health and illness,* ed 5, St Louis, 2014, Saunders.)

to tiny air sacs called *alveoli*. Each lung contains hundreds of millions of alveoli. Accessory structures of the respiratory system include the diaphragm and intercostal muscles (muscles between the ribs). The structural plan of the respiratory system is shown in Figure 7.15. Respiration is controlled by the respiratory control center in the brainstem.

The lungs are paired elastic organs that expand and contract as air moves in and out. Each lung is surrounded by a double membrane called the *pleural sac*. The outer membrane, or parietal pleura, lines the thoracic cavity; the inner membrane, called the visceral pleura, covers the outside of the lung. The pleural cavity is a potential space between the two membranes that contains pleural fluid, which reduces friction between the membranes during breathing. The left lung has an upper lobe and a lower lobe that are separated by an oblique fissure. The right lung has an upper lobe, a lower lobe, and a middle lobe; the three lobes are separated by a horizontal fissure and an oblique fissure. Each lung has a *hilum*, or root, located on the medial surface. The hilum is the space where the bronchi, blood vessels, and nerves enter the lungs.

The respiratory system supplies oxygen to the body and eliminates carbon dioxide. **External respiration** refers to the exchange of gases between the atmosphere and the blood through the alveoli. **Internal respiration** refers to the exchange of gases between the blood and the body cells. The passageways from the nasal cavities down to the alveoli conduct gases to and from the lungs. The upper passageways also serve to warm, filter, and moisten incoming air through mucous membranes and the movement of cilia.

Inhalation requires the contraction of the diaphragm and external intercostal muscles to enlarge the thoracic cavity and draw air into the lungs. Exhalation is a passive process during which the lungs recoil as the respiratory muscles relax and the thorax decreases in size.

Most of the oxygen carried in the blood is bound to hemoglobin in red blood cells. Oxygen is released from hemoglobin as the concentration of oxygen drops in the tissues. Some carbon dioxide is carried on hemoglobin, but most is converted to bicarbonate ion in the blood. Because this reaction also releases hydrogen ions, carbon dioxide is a regulator of blood pH.

HESI Hint

Using the familiar example of an inverted tree, the trachea can be visualized as the trunk and the two primary bronchi and their many subdivisions as the branches. This structure is often referred to as the bronchial tree. The analogy of a bunch of grapes can then be used to explain the terminal components of the respiratory tract, which include the alveolar ducts, alveolar sacs, and alveoli.

Digestive System

The digestive tract is a tube that consists of the mouth, pharynx, esophagus, stomach, small intestine, large intestine, rectum, and anus. The digestive tract has four main layers, from innermost to outer: the mucous membrane, the submucous layer, the muscular layer, and the serous layer. The accessory organs of digestion include the liver, pancreas, and gallbladder. The locations of the digestive organs are seen in Figure 7.16.

Food is ingested into the mouth where it is mechanically broken down by the teeth and tongue in the process of mastication (chewing). Saliva, produced by the three pairs of salivary glands, lubricates and dilutes the chewed food. Saliva contains an enzyme called amylase that starts the digestion of complex carbohydrates. A ball of food called a *bolus* is formed; swallowing forces it into the esophagus. The esophagus is a narrow tube leading from the pharynx to the stomach.

Food enters the stomach where gastric glands secrete hydrochloric acid that unwinds proteins so that the enzyme pepsin can digest them. The layers of muscle in the stomach wall churn and mix the bolus of food with gastric secretions, turning the mass into a soupy substance called *chyme*, which enters the small intestine.

The majority of digestion and absorption of food occurs in the small intestine. The small intestine consists of three major regions: the duodenum, the jejunum, and the ileum. Bile, made by the liver and stored in the gallbladder, empties into the small intestine to emulsify fats. Secretions from the pancreas buffer the acidic chyme from the stomach and contain enzymes such as lipase that digests fats, amylase that continues carbohydrate digestion, and protein-digesting enzymes. The small intestine also secretes protein-digesting enzymes and other enzymes that finish digesting carbohydrates into monosaccharides.

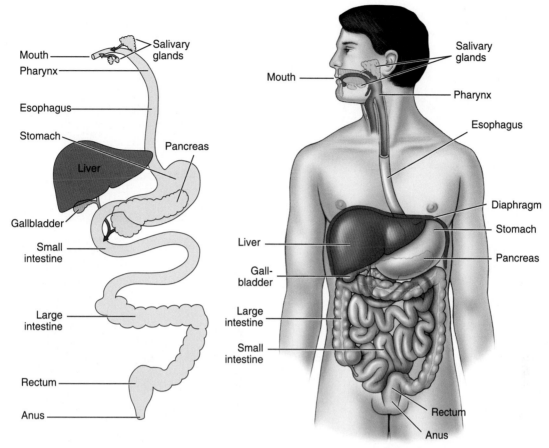

FIGURE 7.16 Location of the digestive organs. (From Herlihy B: *The human body in health and illness*, ed 5, St Louis, 2014, Saunders.)

After digestion, nutrients are absorbed through the walls of the small intestine. The intestinal *villi* are small finger-like projections that greatly increase the surface area for absorption. Amino acids and monosaccharides derived from proteins and carbohydrates are absorbed directly into the blood. Most of the fats are absorbed into the lymph *lacteals*; eventually the fats are added to the bloodstream. The blood from the intestines enters the hepatic portal vein to be routed to the liver for decontamination, so nutrients can be processed before entering the systemic circulation.

The large intestine reabsorbs water and stores and eliminates undigested food. Here also are abundant bacteria, the intestinal (normal) flora. The large intestine is arranged into five portions: the ascending colon, the transverse colon, the descending colon, the sigmoid colon, and the rectum. The opening for defecation (expelling of feces) is the anus.

HESI Hint

During mastication, the teeth reduce ingested food material to smaller particles to increase surface area for chemical digestion. The muscular movements of the stomach and intestines also result in mechanical breakdown of food, thus increasing surface area for digestion.

Urinary System

The urinary system consists of two kidneys, two ureters, the urinary bladder, and the urethra. The kidneys remove wastes and excess water from the body. The ureters are tubes that transport urine from the kidneys to the urinary bladder where urine is temporarily stored. When urination occurs, urine passes from the bladder through the urethra and is eliminated from the body. Locations of urinary system organs are illustrated in Figure 7.17.

Each kidney consists of about one million **nephrons**, which are the functional units of the kidney. The nephron consists of a tubule, a glomerulus, and a glomerular capsule (also called Bowman's capsule). The nephrons filter the blood and form urine in a three-step process. The first step of urine formation is **filtration**, which occurs in the glomerulus. The glomerulus is a network of capillaries surrounded by Bowman's capsule (the glomerulus and Bowman's capsule together are called the *renal corpuscle*). Filtration begins as blood enters the glomerulus under pressure from the renal artery. As blood

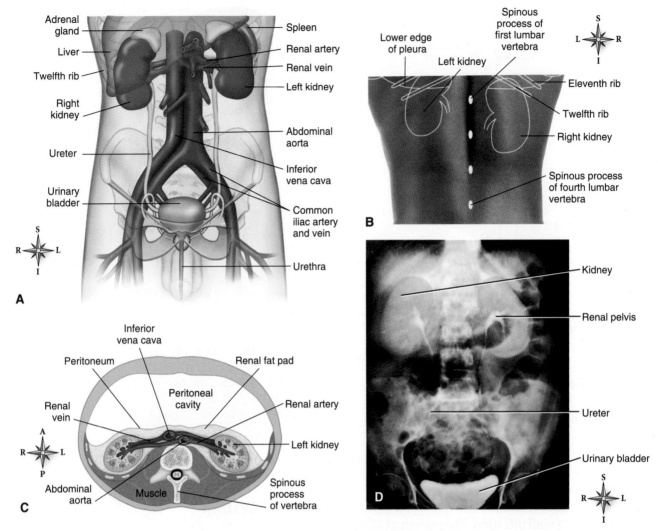

FIGURE 7.17 Location of urinary organs. **A,** Diagram (frontal view). **B,** Posterior body image with palpable landmarks. **C,** Diagram (axial view). **D,** Contrast-enhanced radiograph. (From Patton KT, Thibodeau GA: *Structure & function of the body*, ed 15, St Louis, 2016, Elsevier.)

flows through the glomerulus, water and solutes from the blood plasma are pushed through the capillary wall into Bowman's capsule. The second and third steps of urine formation occur simultaneously. **Reabsorption** occurs as the filtrate exiting Bowman's capsule travels through the tubule. As filtrate passes through the tubule, water and vital nutrients leave the nephron by diffusion and are reabsorbed into the blood. **Secretion** is the process in which substances such as hydrogen ions, nitrogenous wastes, and drugs are secreted from peritubular capillaries and added to the filtrate inside the tubule. The final product of the entire process is urine, which flows into the collecting duct—the last part of the nephron—before the leaving the kidney and flowing down the ureters and into the bladder.

Urine consists of about 95% water and 5% waste products.

HESI Hint

The analogy of a wastewater treatment facility linked to an incredibly efficient recycling center may help explain the big picture of urinary system function. The central role of the kidneys is to serve as regulators of the internal environment. Most chemical exchanges with blood occur in the kidneys where they filter and process the blood to produce urine. In effect, they filter the body fluids of liquid sewage and at the same time retain essential chemicals and nutrients.

Reproductive System

The male and female sex organs (the testes and ovaries) produce gametes (sex cells) through

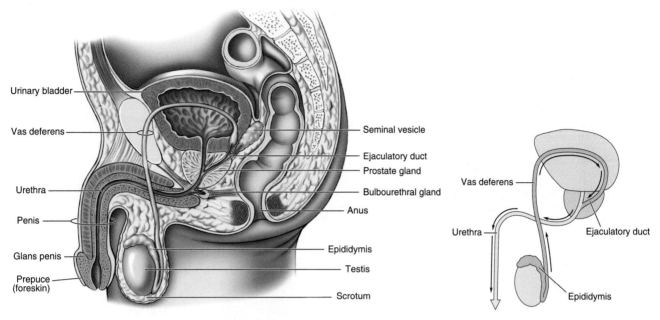

FIGURE 7.18 Male reproductive organs. (From Herlihy B: *The human body in health and illness,* ed 5, St Louis, 2014, Saunders.)

meiosis and also produce hormones. These activities are under the control of tropic hormones from the pituitary gland. Reproductive activity is cyclic in women but continuous in men. Figures 7.18 and 7.19 show the location of male and female reproductive organs.

Male Reproductive System

In males, spermatozoa develop within the seminiferous tubules of each testis. The interstitial cells between the seminiferous tubules produce testosterone. This male hormone influences sperm cell development and also produces the male secondary sex characteristics such as increased facial hair and body hair as well as voice deepening. Once produced, the sperm are matured and stored in the epididymis of each testis. During ejaculation, the pathway for the sperm includes the vas deferens, ejaculatory duct, and urethra. Along the pathway are glands that produce the transport medium or semen. These include the seminal vesicles, prostate gland, and bulbourethral (Cowper's) glands.

Testicular activity is under the control of two anterior pituitary hormones. FSH regulates sperm production. LH stimulates the interstitial cells to produce testosterone.

Female Reproductive System

In females, each month, under the influence of FSH, several eggs ripen within the ovarian follicles. Estrogen produced by the follicle initiates the preparation of the endometrium of the uterus for pregnancy. At approximately day 14 of the cycle, a surge of LH is released from the pituitary gland, which stimulates ovulation and the conversion of the follicle to the corpus luteum. The corpus luteum secretes the hormones progesterone and estrogen, which further stimulate development of the endometrium. After ovulation, the egg (ovum) is swept into the oviduct or fallopian tube. Fertilization, should it occur, happens while the egg is in the oviduct.

If fertilization occurs, the corpus luteum remains functional. If fertilization does not occur, the corpus luteum degenerates and menstruation begins. The fertilized egg, or *zygote*, travels to the uterus and implants itself within the endometrium. In the uterus, the developing embryo is nourished by the placenta, which is formed by maternal and embryonic tissues. During pregnancy, hormones from the placenta maintain the endometrium and prepare the mammary glands for breast milk production.

HESI Hint

To understand the processes involved in the menstrual cycle, first learn the functions of each hormone. Then focus on the specific actions of the hormones while moving through the cycle.

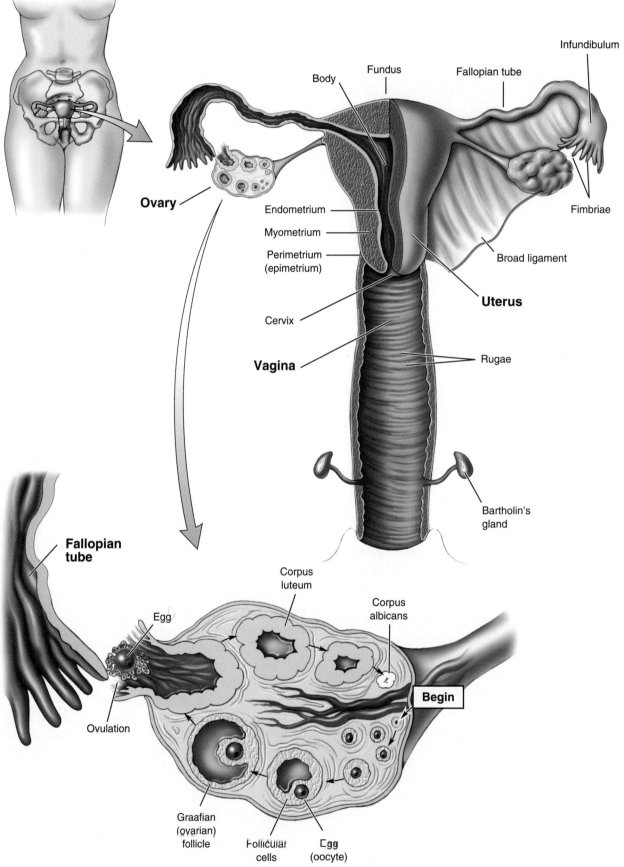

FIGURE 7.19 Female reproductive organs. (From Herlihy B: *The human body in health and illness,* ed 5, St Louis, 2014, Saunders.)

REVIEW QUESTIONS

1. Which term indicates a direction toward the head?
   A. Cranial
   B. Dorsal
   C. Ventral
   D. Caudal

2. Which plane separates the abdominal cavity from the thoracic cavity?
   A. Sagittal
   B. Transverse
   C. Frontal
   D. Oblique

3. Which type of tissue forms the lining of organs?
   A. Nervous
   B. Connective
   C. Muscle
   D. Epithelial

4. What is the name of the outermost layer of skin?
   A. Stratum basale
   B. Stratum corneum
   C. Stratum lucidum
   D. Stratum spinosum

5. What substance protects the skin against radiation from the sun?
   A. Melanin
   B. Keratin
   C. Cytoplasm
   D. Sebum

6. From superior to inferior, the sequence of the vertebral column is:
   A. Sacrum, coccyx, thoracic, lumbar, and cervical
   B. Coccyx, sacrum, lumbar, thoracic, and cervical
   C. Cervical, lumbar, thoracic, sacrum, and coccyx
   D. Cervical, thoracic, lumbar, sacrum, and coccyx

7. What cells are responsible for breaking down bone tissue?
   A. Osteoblasts
   B. Osteocytes
   C. Osteoclasts
   D. Osteogenic cells

8. What cells produce the fibrocartilaginous callus between the two broken ends of a bone?
   A. Osteoblasts and osteoclasts
   B. Fibroblasts and osteoblasts
   C. Osteocytes and osteoclasts
   D. Fibroblasts and osteocytes

9. What protein makes up the thick contractile elements of muscle tissue?
   A. Troponin
   B. Tropomyosin
   C. Actin
   D. Myosin

10. What branch of the nervous system is responsible for voluntary muscle movements?
    A. Somatic
    B. Autonomic
    C. Sympathetic
    D. Parasympathetic

11. What part of a nerve cell transmits impulses to other cells?
    A. Soma
    B. Body
    C. Axon
    D. Dendrite

12. What gland increases calcium levels in the blood?
    A. Pancreas
    B. Parathyroid
    C. Thyroid
    D. Adrenal

13. What chamber of the heart delivers blood to the aorta?
    A. Left atrium
    B. Right ventricle
    C. Right atrium
    D. Left ventricle

14. Which structure prevents food and liquid from entering the lungs?
    A. Trachea
    B. Pharynx
    C. Larynx
    D. Bronchus

15. What organ converts bilirubin into bile?
    A. Small intestine
    B. Liver
    C. Large intestine
    D. Stomach

16. What is the role of luteinizing hormone in the female reproductive system?
    A. Stimulates ovulation
    B. Stimulates egg development
    C. Stimulates the secretion of estrogens
    D. Stimulates development of the endometrium

ANSWERS TO REVIEW QUESTIONS

1. A
2. B
3. D
4. B
5. A
6. D
7. C
8. B
9. D
10. A
11. C
12. B
13. D
14. C
15. B
16. A

POSTTEST

1. Select the correct definition of the underlined word in the sentence.
   The doctor gave a <u>concise</u> explanation of the treatment plan.
   A. Long and confusing
   B. Hasty and incomplete
   C. Strong and forceful
   D. Brief and clear

2. Select the words for the blanks that make this sentence grammatically correct. Sam cooked dinner for _____ and _____.
   A. him, me
   B. him, I
   C. he, I
   D. he, me

3. How does a catalyst increase the rate of a chemical reaction?
   A. By increasing the temperature
   B. By increasing the concentration
   C. By reducing the activation energy
   D. By reducing the surface area

   Change the fraction to a decimal:

4. $5/16 =$ _____
   A. 0.50
   B. 0.60
   C. 0.3125
   D. 0.4165

5. Change the decimal to a percentage: $0.0004 =$
   _____
   A. 0.004%
   B. 0.04%
   C. 0.4%
   D. 4.0%

6. Which word in the sentence is an adverb?
   She suddenly felt as if someone was watching her.

   A. suddenly
   B. felt
   C. was
   D. watching

7. Solve for x: $53 + x = 47$
   A. 100
   B. -100
   C. 6
   D. -6

8. Which word means the same as the underlined words in the sentence?
   If we don't find ways to improve our products, our business will <u>stop developing</u>.
   A. Deteriorate
   B. Migrate
   C. Compensate
   D. Stagnate

9. How many moles of hydrogen fluoride (HF) are needed to balance the following equation?
   $2F_2 + 2H_2O \rightarrow \_HF + O_2$
   A. 4
   B. 3
   C. 2
   D. 1

10. Which sentence contains a proper noun?
    A. We went to the zoo to see the animals.
    B. I've never been to London before.
    C. The mayor arrived in time for the parade.
    D. The general's army traveled south.

11. One length of rope is 3.5 feet long and another is 4.2 feet long. How many feet longer is the second length of rope than the first?
    A. 0.7
    B. 0.8
    C. 1.2
    D. 1.7

12. Which is an imperative sentence?
    A. Oh, I can't believe you did that.
    B. How dare you!
    C. Who do you think you are?
    D. Please go away.

13. Which two types of blood cells are phagocytic?
    A. Neutrophils and macrophages
    B. Eosinophils and erythrocytes
    C. Macrophages and eosinophils
    D. Erythrocytes and neutrophils

14. Select the meaning of the underlined word in the sentence.
    Bob tried to make up for his rude behavior with an _anemic_ apology.
    A. Sincere
    B. Weak
    C. Brief
    D. Lengthy

15. If 4 cups of butter are needed to make 8 cakes, how much butter is needed to make 5 cakes?
    A. 2.25 cups
    B. 2.50 cups
    C. 3.25 cups
    D. 3.50 cups

16. Select the best word for the blank in the following sentence.
    The prize money was divided _____ all the winners.
    A. between
    B. among
    C. throughout
    D. over

17. Multiply $^7/_{18} \times {}^3/_4$ (Reduce the product to the lowest terms.)
    A. $^2/_7$
    B. $^{10}/_{22}$
    C. $^7/_{24}$
    D. $^{28}/_{24}$

18. Chromosomes align across the center of the cell during which phase of mitosis?
    A. Anaphase
    B. Telophase
    C. Metaphase
    D. Prophase

19. Which word means the same as the underlined words in the sentence?
    The oil tycoon amassed an _extremely large_ amount of wealth.
    A. Vital
    B. Residual
    C. Prodigious
    D. Tenuous

20. What mode of transmission spreads infection through tiny respiratory particles?
    A. Droplet
    B. Airborne
    C. Vector
    D. Vehicle

21. Which homeostatic process causes a reaction that reverses the effect of a stimulus?
    A. Catabolism
    B. Anabolism
    C. Positive feedback
    D. Negative feedback

22. Which word in this sentence is an indirect object?
    The manager gave Oscar the keys to the store.
    A. manager
    B. Oscar
    C. keys
    D. store

23. Which sentence includes a euphemism?
    A. Bill had to be let go because he was always late for work.
    B. Dave looked pale as a ghost when he heard the news.
    C. The coach's bark was worse than his bite.
    D. Mom told us to get ready for bed ASAP.

24. What is the end result of DNA translation?
    A. Synthesis of proteins
    B. Formation of a DNA template
    C. Synthesis of mRNA
    D. Formation of identical DNA molecules

25. What determines the mass number of an element?
    A. Mass of protons and electrons
    B. Number of neutrons and electrons
    C. Average mass of an element's isotopes
    D. Number of protons and neutrons

26. What element transports oxygen in the blood?
    A. Potassium
    B. Calcium
    C. Iron
    D. Sodium

27. After making a scientific observation, you develop an explanation. This explanation is tested by performing a repeatable procedure. What is this procedure called?
    A. Hypothesis
    B. Experiment
    C. Conclusion
    D. Theory

28. Which of the following describes an acid?
    A. It changes red litmus paper to blue.
    B. It contains a hydroxyl group.
    C. It donates protons.
    D. It has a pH above 7.

29. The tissue that forms over the site of a broken bone is called a _____.
    A. fracture
    B. clot
    C. callus
    D. hematoma

30. Which of the following sentences is grammatically correct?
    A. We saw dolphins on a boat ride during our trip.
    B. We took a trip to see the dolphins on a boat ride.
    C. We went to see the dolphins on a boat ride.
    D. We went on a boat ride to see the dolphins.

31. What is 60% of 80?
    A. 42
    B. 48
    C. 54
    D. 60

32. What gland produces hormones that regulate the amount of glucose in the blood?
    A. Adrenal
    B. Thyroid
    C. Pituitary
    D. Pancreas

33. Select the meaning of the underlined word in the sentence.
    The boxer could see <u>overt</u> signs of weakness in his opponent.
    A. Obvious
    B. Hidden
    C. Small
    D. Important

34. Muscle contraction is triggered by the release of _____ ions into the muscle cell.
    A. chloride
    B. sodium
    C. calcium
    D. magnesium

35. Select the correct definition for the underlined word in the sentence.
    Paul's passion for writing started to <u>atrophy</u> once he became a successful author.
    A. Weaken
    B. Increase
    C. Improve
    D. Change

36. What happens during an oxidation reaction?
    A. Hydrogen ions are gained
    B. Hydrogen ions are lost
    C. Electrons are gained
    D. Electrons are lost

37. What is the mode in the following data set?
    {2, 4, 4, 4, 5, 6, 6, 9}
    A. 4
    B. 5
    C. 6
    D. 7

38. Where do the pulmonary vessels and bronchi enter the lung?
    A. Larynx
    B. Hilum
    C. Trachea
    D. Pharynx

39. What is 6:30 PM in military time?
    A. 2030
    B. 0630
    C. 1430
    D. 1830

40. Divide: $2\frac{1}{2} \div \frac{5}{6}$
    A. 6
    B. 3
    C. $2\frac{5}{12}$
    D. $2\frac{1}{12}$

41. The somatic nervous system is also known as the _____ nervous system.
    A. involuntary
    B. voluntary
    C. sympathetic
    D. parasympathetic

42. What type of bond involves the complete transfer of electrons from one atom to another?
    A. Ionic
    B. Hydrogen
    C. Polar covalent
    D. Non-polar covalent

43. Which word means *spread out over a large area*?
    A. Profuse
    B. Obtuse
    C. Diffuse
    D. Abstruse

44. Which word means the same as the underlined word in the sentence?
    Despite receiving some benign criticism, the art exhibit was a rousing success.
    A. Foolish
    B. Unwanted
    C. Hurtful
    D. Mild

Use the passage below to answer questions 45–50.

Jonas Salk

Jonas Salk was an American physician and one of the leading medical researchers of the twentieth century. He is famous for creating the first safe and effective vaccine for polio, a highly infectious incurable disease that was responsible for thousands of cases of paralysis each year in the United States.

Salk received degrees in science and medicine before serving as director of the Virus Research Laboratory at the University of Pittsburgh in 1947. By this time, polio was one of the most feared diseases of the twentieth century. Polio, which is caused by the poliovirus, can cause paralysis of muscles in the limbs, throat, and chest. Polio can lead to death when the muscles responsible for breathing become paralyzed.

By 1951, Salk developed a vaccine made of "killed" poliovirus. The vaccine was produced from polioviruses that had been grown in a laboratory and then destroyed. When the "killed" virus was injected into the bloodstream, Salk reasoned that the vaccine would trick the immune system into producing anti-polio antibodies. Salk also believed his vaccine would immunize patients without risking infection.

Early testing of the Salk vaccine began in 1952, when children at two institutions were injected with the vaccine. In 1954, about 650,000 children received the Salk vaccine or a placebo. All of the test subjects who received the vaccine developed anti-polio antibodies and did not experience any significant negative reactions to the vaccine. Within two years of the vaccine's approval, cases of polio had fallen by almost 90%. Since 1979, no new cases of polio have been reported in the United States.

By the time the vaccine was approved for use, Jonas Salk was considered a national hero. In 1955, he received a special citation from President Dwight D. Eisenhower at a ceremony held in the Rose Garden at the White House. Having developed the vaccine that would eradicate polio in the United States, Salk will always be remembered as one of the greatest medical pioneers of the twentieth century.

45. Which is the best summary of the passage?
    A. Jonas Salk created the first successful polio vaccine. He developed a vaccine made of "killed" poliovirus. After the vaccine was approved for public use, the number of new cases of polio began to decline rapidly. Salk was considered a national hero for stopping polio.
    B. Jonas Salk created the first safe and effective polio vaccine. He tested the vaccine by injecting live poliovirus into his test subjects. Within a few years of the vaccine's approval, the number of polio cases had decreased dramatically. Today he is known as the man who cured polio.
    C. Jonas Salk was a famous medical researcher. He discovered the poliovirus in 1947 and began working on a cure. By 1951, he developed a vaccine that was able to trick the body into developing antibodies to kill the virus. When the vaccine was approved, Salk became famous.

D. Jonas Salk was a famous American physician who created a vaccine for the poliovirus. In 1952, the vaccine was tested on children with polio. All the children developed antibodies and were cured of polio. He became a hero for ending polio in the United States.

46. Which is not a detail from the passage?
   A. Salk was the director of a virus research laboratory in Pittsburgh.
   B. Salk received a citation from the President of the United States.
   C. Salk discovered the poliovirus at his laboratory in 1947.
   D. Salk received degrees in both science and medicine.

47. What is the purpose of the polio vaccine?
   A. To help reduce the symptoms of polio
   B. To make people immune to the poliovirus
   C. To destroy the poliovirus within the body
   D. To cure people suffering from polio

48. According to the passage, why was Jonas Salk considered a national hero?
   A. He discovered the poliovirus.
   B. He created a vaccine for polio.
   C. He developed a cure for polio.
   D. He founded a polio research laboratory.

49. What is the main purpose of the passage?
   A. To explain why Jonas Salk is an important figure
   B. To educate the reader about vaccine science
   C. To describe the effects of polio on the body
   D. To encourage people to receive the polio vaccine

50. What does the word *eradicate* mean as it is used in the last paragraph?
   A. To decrease in severity
   B. To decrease in size
   C. To completely destroy
   D. To completely control

ANSWERS TO POSTTEST

1. D—*Concise* means "brief and clearly stated."
2. A—Objective case pronouns are required to complete this sentence. The pronouns "him" and "me" are objects of the preposition "for."
3. C—A catalyst accelerates a reaction by reducing the activation energy, which is the amount of energy necessary for a reaction to occur.
4. C—To convert $^5/_{16}$ to a decimal, change the fraction into a division problem:

   $$
   \begin{array}{r}
   0.3125 \\
   16)\overline{5.0000} \\
   -\underline{48}\downarrow\downarrow\downarrow \quad (16 \times 3 = 48) \\
   20\downarrow\downarrow \\
   -\underline{16}\downarrow\downarrow \quad (16 \times 1 = 16) \\
   40\downarrow \\
   -\underline{32}\downarrow \quad (16 \times 2 = 32) \\
   80 \\
   -\underline{80} \quad (16 \times 5 = 80) \\
   0
   \end{array}
   $$

   $^5/_{16} = 0.3125$
5. B—To change a decimal to a percentage, move the decimal point two places to the right. Insert the percent sign after the new number: $0.0004 = 0.04\%$
6. A—An adverb is a word or phrase that modifies a verb, an adjective, or another adverb. In this sentence, the adverb "suddenly" modifies the verb "felt."
7. D—Solve for x: $53 + x = 47$
   Isolate the variable (subtract 53 from both sides):
   $53 - 53 + x = 47 - 53$
   $x = -6$
8. D—*Stagnate* means to stop developing or progressing.
9. A—Four moles of hydrogen fluoride are needed to balance the following equation:
   $2F_2 + 2H_2O \rightarrow \_HF + O_2$
   The left side of the equation consists of 4 fluorine atoms, 4 hydrogen atoms, and 2 oxygen atoms. The following reaction will result in the same number of fluorine, hydrogen, and oxygen atoms on the right side of the equation:
   $2F_2 + 2H_2O \rightarrow 4HF + O_2$

10. B—A proper noun is the official name of a person, place, or thing. London is a proper noun.

11. A—If the first rope is 3.5 feet long and the second rope is 4.2 feet long, the second rope is 0.7 feet longer than the first:

$$\begin{array}{r} 4.2 \\ -\ 3.5 \\ \hline 0.7 \end{array}$$

12. D—An imperative sentence makes a command or request. *Please go away* is an example of an imperative sentence.

13. A—Neutrophils and macrophages are phagocytic white blood cells. Both types of cells destroy invading pathogens and therefore play a key role in the innate immune response.

14. B—In this sentence, *anemic* means "weak."

15. B—If 4 cups of butter are needed to make 8 cakes, the amount of butter to make 5 cakes can be calculated using the following proportion:
4 cups : 8 cakes :: x cups : 5 cakes
Rewrite the ratios as fractions:
$^4/_8 = {}^x/_5$
Multiply the diagonal numbers:
$4 \times 5 = 20$
Divide the product (20) by the remaining number (8):
$20 \div 8 = 2.5$
$x = 2.5$ cups

16. B—*Among* is used to show a relationship involving more than two persons or things that are part of a group. In this sentence, the indefinite pronoun *all* implies more than two winners.

17. C—Solve: $^7/_{18} \times {}^3/_4$
Multiply the numerators together: $7 \times 3 = 21$
Multiply the denominators together: $18 \times 4 = 72$
Find the greatest common factor of 21 and 72, then divide the numerator and the denominator by this number:
21: 1, 3, 7, 21
72: 1, 2, 3, 4, 6, 8, 9, 12, 18, 24, 36, 72
$21 \div 3 = 7$
$72 \div 3 = 24$
Solution:
$^{21}/_{72} = {}^7/_{24}$

18. C—During metaphase, the chromosomes align along what is called the metaphase plate or the center of the cell.

19. C—*Prodigious* means "extremely large in amount or size."

20. B—Airborne transmission refers to the spread of infection through tiny respiratory particles that remain suspended in the air for an extended time.

21. D—Homeostasis refers to the tendency of the body to maintain a stable internal environment. Homeostasis is maintained through negative feedback loops. Negative feedback is a response to a stimulus that reverses the effects of the original stimulus in order to return the system to its original state.

22. B—An indirect object is a person or thing that is indirectly affected by the action of the verb. Indirect objects are located between the verb and the direct object. In this sentence, the indirect object "Oscar" is located between the verb "gave" and the direct object "keys."

23. A—A euphemism is a mild, indirect, or vague term or phrase that replaces another term or phrase that is considered harsh or offensive. In this sentence, "let go" is a euphemism for "fired."

24. A—Translation is the process by which genetic information from mRNA is used to make proteins.

25. D—Mass number is the combined number of protons and neutrons in an element.

26. C—Hemoglobin is a protein that carries oxygen in red blood cells. Oxygen binds to the iron atom of the heme group and is transported throughout the body.

27. B—An *experiment* is a repeatable procedure of gathering data to test an explanation (hypothesis).

28. C—An acid is a compound that donates a proton (H^+) in an acid-base reaction.

29. C—During bone healing, chondrocytes and osteoblasts form a soft *callus* that connects and stabilizes the broken bone. As cartilage is absorbed and replaced by bone tissue, the soft callus is remodeled into a hard callus.

30. D—Misplaced modifiers are single words or groups of words that are incorrectly separated from the words they are intended to modify. In this example, the phrase "on a boat ride" belongs closest to the word it modifies (*we*).

31. B—60% of 80 is 48. The answer may be calculated using the percent formula:
$$\frac{Part}{Whole} = \frac{\%}{100}$$
$$\frac{x}{80} = \frac{60}{100}$$

Multiply the diagonal numbers together:
$80 \times 60 = 4800$
Divide by the remaining number:
$4800 \div 100 = 48$

32. D—The pancreas secretes insulin and glucagon, which are hormones that regulate blood glucose levels.

33. A—*Overt* is an adjective meaning "obvious or easily observed."

34. C—Muscle contraction, which is regulated by the troponin-tropomyosin complex, is triggered by the release of calcium ions in the muscle cell.

35. A—In this sentence, *atrophy* is a verb that means "to become weaker."

36. D—Oxidation-reduction (redox) reactions involve the transfer of electrons. Oxidation involves the loss of electrons.

37. A—The mode is the most frequently occurring number in a set of values. The mode of the following data set is 4:
{2, 4, 4, 4, 5, 6, 6, 9}

38. B—The hilum is the opening at the medial aspect of each lung. Blood vessels, nerves, and bronchi enter the lung through the hilum.

39. D—Military time uses the numbers 00 to 23 to represent the hours in a 24-hour day. Times after 12 pm are converted to military time by adding 12 to the hour number (minutes remain the same): 6:30 PM + 12 = 1830 hours

40. B—Solve: $2\frac{1}{2} \div \frac{5}{6}$
First, convert the mixed number to an improper fraction:
$2\frac{1}{2} = \frac{5}{2}$
To divide by a fraction, invert the second fraction and multiply:
$\frac{5}{2} \div \frac{5}{6} = \frac{5}{2} \times \frac{6}{5}$
Calculate the product by multiplying the numerators together and the denominators together:
$\frac{5}{2} \times \frac{6}{5} = \frac{30}{10}$

Find the greatest common factor of 30 and 10, then divide the numerator and the denominator by this number:
30: 1, 2, 5, 6, 10
10: 1, 2, 5, 10
$30 \div 10 = 3$
$10 \div 10 = 1$
Solution: $\frac{30}{10} = \frac{3}{1} = 3$

41. B—The somatic nervous system is also called the voluntary nervous system because it controls voluntary muscle movements.

42. A—Ionic bonds are formed by the complete transfer of one or more outer electrons to form a neutral compound.

43. C—*Diffuse* means "spread out over a large area."

44. D—*Benign* means "mild; harmless."

45. A—This summary includes all of the main ideas of the passage: Jonas Salk created the first successful polio vaccine; he developed a vaccine made of "killed" poliovirus; the number of new cases of polio began to decline rapidly after the vaccine was approved; Salk was considered a national hero for stopping polio.

46. C—The poliovirus was discovered in 1908. Salk did not discover the poliovirus.

47. B—The purpose of the polio vaccine was to make people immune to the poliovirus.

48. B—Salk was considered a national hero because he developed a safe and highly effective polio vaccine.

49. A—The main purpose of the passage is to explain why Jonas Salk is an important historical figure.

50. C—The passage states that no new cases of polio have been reported in the United States since 1979. From this information, the reader can deduce that *eradicate* means "completely destroy."

GLOSSARY

A

Abstract noun The name of a quality or a general idea (e.g., bravery, democracy).

Acetylcholine A neurotransmitter that binds to receptors on the outside of the muscle fiber and initiates depolarization within the sarcolemma.

Acid A compound that is a hydrogen or proton donor. Acids corrode metals, denature proteins, change blue litmus paper red, and become less acidic when mixed with bases.

Action potential An impulse generated by the nervous system and transmitted along the axon of a nerve cell.

Active transport The movement of molecules against a concentration gradient (i.e., from a region of lower concentration to a region of higher concentration) that requires an expenditure of energy.

Adaptive immune system The body's second line of defense against infection; a slower-acting immune response consisting of specialized cells that identify and destroy specific pathogens.

Adjective A word, phrase, or clause that modifies a noun (the *biology* book) or pronoun (He is *nice*).

Adverb A word, phrase, or clause that modifies a verb, an adjective, or another adverb.

Alleles Alternate versions of a gene.

Amino acids Organic compounds that contain at least one amino group and a carboxyl group; the building blocks of proteins.

Anatomical position Provides a baseline reference point for areas of the body. In this position, the body is erect, the feet are slightly apart, the arms are at the sides, and the palms of the hands are facing forward.

Anterior (Ventral) Directional term meaning *toward the front*.

Anticodon A group of three nucleotides on a tRNA molecule that corresponds with the complementary codon of an mRNA molecule.

Antonym A word that means the opposite of another word.

Appendicular skeleton The part of the skeleton that includes the shoulder girdles, the hip girdles, and the extremities.

Assumption A set of beliefs that the writer has about the subject.

Atom The basic building block of matter; contains a nucleus with protons and neutrons surrounded by one or more electrons.

Atomic number The number of protons in the nucleus; defines an atom of a particular element.

Atomic weight The average mass of all the isotopes of an element.

Autonomic nervous system Division of the peripheral nervous system that regulates digestion, blood pressure, the diameter of blood vessels, and the force and rate of heart muscle contraction. The two divisions of the autonomic nervous system are the *parasympathetic division* ("rest and digest") and the *sympathetic division* ("fight or flight").

Axial skeleton Consists of the skull, vertebral column, twelve pairs of ribs, and sternum.

B

Base A hydrogen or proton acceptor; generally has a hydroxide (OH⁻) group in the makeup of the molecule. Also called *alkaline compounds*, bases are substances that denature proteins, making them feel very slick. They change red litmus paper blue and become less basic when mixed with acids.

Basic unit of measure Standard unit of a system by which a quantity is accounted for and expressed (grams, liters, or meters).

Binary fission Type of asexual reproduction in which the parent cell splits into two identical daughter cells.

Biochemistry The study of chemical processes in living organisms.

Body planes Imaginary lines that divide the body at certain angles. Types of body planes include sagittal, midsagittal, frontal (coronal), and transverse (horizontal).

Brainstem Part of the brain that is continuous with the spinal cord; consists of the midbrain, pons, and medulla oblongata; controls many vital functions such as respiration and heart rate.

C

Catalysts Substances that accelerate a reaction by reducing the activation energy, which is the amount of energy necessary for a reaction to occur.

Caudal Located or directed *away from the head*.

Cells The basic units of life and the building blocks of tissues and organs.

Celsius A temperature system used in most of the world and by the scientific community; abbreviated °C. It has these characteristics: zero degrees (0°C) is the freezing point of pure water at sea level, and 100°C is the boiling point of pure water at sea level. The average normal body temperature is 37°C.

Cerebellum The part of the brain responsible for muscular coordination.

Cerebrum The part of the brain associated with sensory interpretation, movement, thinking, and personality.

Chain of infection The six steps (or links) that describe how an infectious agent enters a susceptible host.

Chemical equations The visual representation of a chemical reaction. Equations are expressed with reactants on the left side and products on the right side: Reactants → Products; Reactants ← Products; Reactants ↔ Products.

Chromosomes Compact, linear-shaped bodies located within the nucleus of a cell; strands of DNA.

Citric acid cycle (also called Krebs cycle) Series of reactions occurring in the mitochondrial matrix during cellular respiration.

Clause A group of words that has a subject and a predicate.

Cliché An expression or idea that has lost its originality or impact over time because of excessive use.

Codon Three-base sequence of messenger RNA.

Collective noun A noun that represents a group of persons, animals, or things (e.g., family, flock, furniture).

Combustion A self-sustaining exothermic chemical reaction; usually initiated by heat acting on oxygen and a fuel compound such as hydrocarbons.

Common denominator A number that is divisible by all the denominators of a group of fractions.

Common noun The general, not the particular, name of a person, place, or thing (e.g., dog, house, baseball).

Compound A combination of two or more elements or atoms.

Compound sentence A sentence that has two or more independent clauses. Each independent clause has a subject and a predicate and can stand alone as a sentence.

Concentration gradient The difference in concentrations of a substance across a membrane.

Conjunction A word that links two words, phrases, or clauses.

Connotation The emotions or feelings that the reader attaches to words.

Constant A number or value in a mathematical expression that does not change.

Context clue The information surrounding an unknown word or words that provides insight as to the meaning of those words.

Contralateral Located or occurring on the *opposite side* of the body.

Covalent bond A chemical bond formed by the equal sharing of electrons between atoms.

Cranial Located or directed *toward the head*.

Cytokinesis The final phase of the cell cycle (after interphase and mitosis); the process during which the cytoplasm of the parent cell divides into two new daughter cells.

D

Declarative A sentence that makes a statement.

Decomposition The breakdown of a compound into its component parts; often described as the opposite of a synthesis reaction.

Deep Directional term meaning *further into* the body.

Denominator The bottom number in a fraction.

Deoxyribonucleic acid (DNA) A double helical structure with a backbone of alternating sugar and phosphate groups. Each DNA molecule contains the unique genetic code for an organism.

Deoxyribose A sugar used in the formation of DNA.

Dependent clause A clause that begins with a subordinating conjunction and does not express a complete thought and therefore cannot stand alone as a sentence.

Dermis Deep layer of skin; consists of connective tissue with blood vessels, nerve endings, and associated skin structures.

Diencephalon The part of the brain that contains the thalamus, which routes incoming sensory information to the appropriate part of the cerebrum; and the hypothalamus, which monitors many of the conditions of the body, controls the autonomic nervous system, and interacts with the endocrine system.

Digit Any number from 0 through 9.

Direct object The person or thing that is directly affected by the action of the verb.

Distal Directional term meaning *farther away* from a point of reference or attachment.

Dividend The number being divided.

Divisor The number by which the dividend is divided.

Double replacement A reaction that involves two ionic compounds. The positive ion from one compound combines with the negative ion of the other compound. The result is two new ionic compounds that have "switched partners."

E

Electron A subatomic particle located at the outermost part of the atom; a negatively charged particle. Electrons orbit the nucleus at fantastic speeds, forming electron clouds.

Electron clouds Another name for atomic orbitals; areas around the nucleus where electrons are believed to be present.

Electron transport chain A series of steps in cellular respiration that produces water and ATP.

Endocardium The inner layer of the heart; forms the inner lining of the four chambers and covers the heart valves.

Endosteum Thin vascular layer of connective tissue that lines the medullary cavities of bones.

Epidermis Superficial layer of skin made of dead, keratinized epithelial cells.

Equilibrium A state in which reactants are forming products at the same rate that products are forming reactants.

Erythrocytes Red blood cells.

Euphemism A mild, indirect, or vague term that has been substituted for one that is considered harsh, blunt, or offensive.

Exclamatory A sentence expressing strong feelings or making an exclamation.

Exponent A number or symbol placed above and after another number or symbol (i.e., a superscript); indicates the number of times to multiply.

Expression A mathematic sentence containing constants and variables (e.g., $3x - 2$).

External respiration The exchange of gases between the atmosphere and the blood through the alveoli.

F

Factor A number that divides evenly into another number.

Fahrenheit A temperature-measuring system used only in the United States, its territories, Belize, and Jamaica; abbreviated °F. It is rarely used for any scientific measurements except for body temperature. It has these characteristics: zero degrees (0°) is the freezing point of sea water or heavy brine at sea level; 32°F is the freezing point of pure water at sea level; 212°F is the boiling point of pure water at sea level inaccurate statement.

Filtration The first step in urine formation; takes place in the glomerulus of the nephron, where excess water and solutes are removed from the blood.

Fraction bar The line between the numerator and denominator; another symbol for division.

G

Genes The basic units of heredity; sections of a DNA strand that code for specific proteins.

Germ theory The theory that infectious diseases are caused by living or nonliving microorganisms.

Glycolysis Anaerobic breakdown of glucose; the first stage in cell respiration.

Golgi apparatus Cell organelle that packages, processes, and distributes molecules inside or outside the cell.

Groups Elements arranged in columns within the periodic table.

H

Hemopoiesis Blood cell formation.

Heterozygous Describes a trait in an organism that contains different alleles.

Histology The study of tissues.

Homeostasis An organism's ability to adjust to external changes while maintaining a relatively stable internal environment.

Homozygous Describes a trait in an organism that contains identical alleles.

I

Imperative A sentence that makes a command or request.

Improper Fraction A fraction with a numerator that is larger than the denominator.

Independent clause A clause that expresses a complete thought and can stand alone as a sentence.

Indirect object The person or thing that is indirectly affected by the action of the verb.

Inference An educated guess or conclusion drawn by the reader based on the available facts and information.

Inferior Directional term meaning *below*.

Innate immune system The body's first line of defense against infection; a rapid response system consisting of physical barriers and inflammatory responses that prevents the spread of pathogens.

Interjection A word or phrase that expresses emotion or exclamation.

Internal respiration The exchange of gases between the blood and the body cells.

Interphase Stage of the cell cycle during which cell growth and DNA synthesis occur.

Interrogative A sentence that asks a question.

Ionic bond An electrostatic attraction between two oppositely charged ions. This type of bond is generally formed between a metal (cation) and a nonmetal (anion).

Ipsilateral Located or occurring on the *same side* of the body.

Isotopes Different forms of the same atom that vary in weight. For a given element, the number of protons remains the same, while the number of neutrons varies to make the different isotopes.

K

Kelvin A unit of measure for temperature that is used only in the scientific community; abbreviated K. It has these characteristics: zero Kelvin (0K) is −273°C and is thought to be the lowest temperature achievable (known as *absolute zero*); the freezing point of water is 273K; the boiling point of water is 373K. The average normal body temperature is 310K.

L

Lateral Directional term meaning *away from the midline.*

Least common denominator The smallest multiple that two numbers share.

Leukocytes White blood cells.

M

Mass number The combined number of protons and neutrons in an element.

Mathematic sign A symbol used in mathematics; makes up one of the three parts of scientific notation and designates whether the number is positive or negative (+ or −).

Mean The sum of all the values in a data set divided by the number of values; often called the *average.*

Medial Directional term meaning *toward the midline.*

Median The middle number of a data set arranged in numerical order.

Meiosis Type of cell division that takes place in the gonads (ovaries and testes) as part of sexual reproduction. In this process, the chromosome number is reduced from 46 to 23, so when the egg and the sperm unite in fertilization, the zygote will have the correct number of chromosomes.

Messenger RNA (mRNA) Type of RNA formed from a template of DNA; carries coded information to form proteins.

Metabolic pathway A series of linked chemical reactions.

Metaphase plate An imaginary line along the middle of the cell where chromosomes line up during metaphase; also called the *equatorial plate.*

Misplaced modifiers Words or groups of words that are not located properly in relation to the words they modify.

Mitosis The phase of the cell cycle in which the parent cell's DNA is duplicated and distributed evenly between two identical daughter cells. Phases of mitosis include prophase, metaphase, anaphase, and telophase.

Mixed Number A whole number combined with a proper fraction.

Mode The number that appears most often in a data set.

Mole Standard unit for expressing the amount of a substance; equal to 6.02×10^{23} units (also known as Avogadro's number).

Myocardium Cardiac muscle tissue that forms the middle layer of the heart.

Myofibrils The basic units of a muscle fiber.

N

Negative feedback A mechanism that reduces the effects of a stimulus and returns a system back to its set point.

Nephrons The functional units of the kidneys that filter wastes out of the blood.

Neuroglia Connective tissue cells that support neurons.

Neurons Nerve cells; the functional units of the nervous system that initiate and conduct impulses to the brain and other parts of the body.

Neutron A subatomic particle that is located in the nucleus of an atom and has no electrical charge.

Noun A word or group of words that names a person, place, thing, or idea.

Nucleus The positively charged mass within an atom. The nucleus is composed of neutrons and protons; it contains nearly all the mass of an atom but occupies only a tiny percentage of the volume.

Numerator The top number in a fraction.

O

Orbit The outermost part of the atom; the fixed path along which an electron spins around the nucleus.

Organelles "Little organs" within a cell that perform specific functions.

Osteoblasts Cells that form bone tissue.

Osteoclasts Cells that break down bone tissue.

Osteocytes Mature bone cells.

Osteogenic cells Undifferentiated bone cells; the only bone cells capable of dividing.

P

Participial phrase A phrase formed by a participle, its object, and the object's modifiers; functions as an adjective.

Participle A type of verb form that functions as an adjective.

Passive Transport The movement of molecules along a concentration gradient (i.e., from a region of high concentration to a region of low concentration) and without the use of energy.

Percent Per hundred (part per hundred).

Pericardium Fluid-filled sac that surrounds the heart.

Periodic table A table that organizes the elements based on their structure and helps predict the properties of each of the elements. It is made up of a series of rows called *periods* and columns called *groups.*

Periods Elements arranged in rows within the periodic table.

Periosteum Fibrous membrane that covers the bones.

Personal pronoun A pronoun that refers to a specific person, place, thing, or idea by indicating the person speaking (first person), the person or people spoken to (second person), or any other person, place, thing, or idea being talked about (third person).

pH The concentrations of acids. The pH scale commonly in use ranges from 0 to 14 and measures the acidity or alkalinity of a solution.

Phagocytosis Process in which cells engulf other cells or food particles through the cell membrane.

Phospholipids Phosphate-containing fat molecules that form the bilayer of a cell membrane.

Photosynthesis Chemical process that converts light energy to synthesize carbohydrates.

Phrase A group of two or more words that acts as a single part of speech in a sentence.

Place value The value of the position of a digit in a number (e.g., in the number 659, the number 5 is in the "tens" position).

Positive feedback A mechanism that increases the effects of an initial stimulus, pushing a system further away from its set point.

Possessive pronoun A form of personal pronoun that shows possession or ownership.

Posterior (dorsal) Directional term meaning *toward the back*.

Predicate The part of a sentence that tells what the subject does or what is done to the subject.

Predicate adjective An adjective that follows a linking verb and helps to explain the subject.

Predicate nominative A noun or pronoun that follows a linking verb and helps to explain or rename the subject.

Prefix A quantifier of metric units. Metric prefixes indicate powers of ten and are situated at the beginning of a metric unit (e.g., "kilogram," where "kilo" is the prefix and "gram" is the basic unit of measure). A given prefix has the same value regardless of which basic unit of measurement (grams, liters, or meters) it precedes.

Preposition A word that shows the relationship of a noun or pronoun to some other word in the sentence.

Product The answer to a multiplication problem.

Products Substances or compounds created from a chemical reaction.

Pronoun A word that takes the place of a noun, another pronoun, or a group of words acting as a noun.

Proper fraction A fraction with a numerator that is smaller than the denominator.

Proper noun The official name of a person, place, or thing (e.g., Fred, Paris, Washington University). Proper nouns are capitalized.

Proportion Two ratios that have equal values.

Proton A subatomic particle that is located in the nucleus of an atom and has a positive electrical charge.

Proximal Directional term meaning *closer to* a point of reference or attachment.

Punnett square Grid used to predict genotype and phenotype of the offspring of sexual reproduction.

Q

Quotient The answer to a division problem.

R

Ratio A relationship between two numbers.

Reabsorption The second step in urine formation; the process that moves water and vital nutrients out of the filtrate and back into the bloodstream.

Reactants Substances that undergo change in a chemical reaction.

Reciprocals Pairs of numbers that equal 1 when multiplied together.

Remainder The portion of the dividend that is not evenly divisible by the divisor.

Remodeling The process of replacing old or damaged bone with new bone.

Ribonucleic acid (RNA) Nucleic acid found in both the nucleus and cytoplasm of the cell; occurs in three forms: mRNA, ribosomal RNA, and tRNA.

Ribose Sugar used in the formation of RNA.

Rough ER Section of the endoplasmic reticulum (ER) that is covered with ribosomes; responsible for protein synthesis and membrane production.

Run-on sentence Grammatical error in which two or more complete sentences are written as though they were one sentence.

S

Saltatory conduction The propagation of an action potential along a myelinated axon from one node of Ranvier to the next.

Sarcolemma The muscle cell membrane.

Sarcomere The smallest functional unit of striated muscle tissue; composed of thick and thin myofibrils.

Sarcoplasmic reticulum A membrane-bound organelle in muscle cells that regulates the calcium ion concentration within the cell.

Scientific notation The scientific system of writing numbers; a method to write very big or very small numbers easily; composed of three parts: a mathematic sign (+ or −), the significand, and the exponential (sometimes called the *logarithm*).

Secretion The third step in urine formation; the process in which ions, waste products, and drugs are secreted back into the renal tubule from the peritubular capillaries.

Sentence A group of words that expresses a complete thought.

Sentence fragment An incomplete sentence.

Sexist language Spoken or written styles that unnecessarily identify gender.

Significand The base value of the number or the value of the number when all the values of ten are removed. Used in scientific notation.

Single replacement Reactions that consist of a more active metal reacting with an ionic compound containing a less active metal to produce a new compound.

Sliding filament model Mechanism of muscle contraction in which myosin binds to actin and pulls it toward the center of the sarcomere.

Smooth ER Section of the endoplasmic reticulum (ER) that lacks ribosomes; functions in detoxification and metabolism of multiple molecules.

Solute The part of a solution that is being dissolved.

Solution A homogeneous mixture of two or more substances.

Solvent The part of the solution that dissolves a solute.

Stop codon Sequence of bases that terminates translation during protein synthesis.

Subject A word, phrase, or clause that names whom or what the sentence is about.

Superficial Directional term meaning *closer to the surface* of the body.

Superior Directional term meaning *above*.

Synonym A word that means the same as another word.

Synthesis A type of chemical reaction in which two or more simple reactants combine to form a single product.

T

Terminating decimal A decimal that is not continuous.

Textspeak A language that is often used in text messages, emails, and other forms of electronic communication; consists of abbreviations, slang, emoticons, and acronyms.

Thrombocytes Platelets.

Tone The attitude or feelings the author expresses about the topic.

Transcription Process during protein synthesis in which the DNA molecule is used as a template to form mRNA.

Transfer RNA (tRNA) An RNA molecule involved in protein synthesis; transfers a specific amino acid to the ribosome and binds it to mRNA.

Translation The process by which genetic information from mRNA is used to make proteins.

Troponin-tropomyosin complex A protein complex on the actin filament that regulates the availability of binding sites for myosin.

V

Variable A letter representing an unknown quantity (e.g., x).

Verb A word or phrase used to express an action or a state of being.

INDEX

Note: Page numbers followed by "b", "t", and "f" refer to boxes, tables, and figures respectively.